INTERVENTIONAL CARDIOLOGY CLINICS

www.interventional.theclinics.com

Editor-in-Chief

MATTHEW J. PRICE

Endovascular Treatment of Peripheral Artery Disease and Critical Limb Ischemia

April 2017 • Volume 6 • Number 2

Editor

EHRIN J. ARMSTRONG

ELSEVIER

1600 John F. Kennedy Boulevard • Suite 1800 • Philadelphia, Pennsylvania, 19103-2899

http://www.theclinics.com

INTERVENTIONAL CARDIOLOGY CLINICS Volume 6, Number 2
April 2017 ISSN 2211-7458, ISBN-13: 978-0-323-52413-1

Editor: Lauren Boyle
Developmental Editor: Susan Showalter

Interventional Cardiology Clinics (ISSN 2211-7458) is published quarterly by Elsevier Inc., 360 Park Avenue South, New York, NY 10010-1710. Months of issue are January, April, July, and October. Subscription prices are USD 195 per year for US individuals, USD 449 for US institutions, USD 100 per year for US students, USD 195 per year for Canadian individuals, USD 536 for Canadian institutions, USD 150 per year for Canadian students, USD 295 per year for international individuals, USD 536 for international institutions, and USD 150 per year for international students. To receive student/resident rate, orders must be accompanied by name of affiliated institution, date of term, and the *signature* of program/residency coordinator on institution letterhead. Orders will be billed at individual rate until proof of status is received. Foreign air speed delivery is included in all *Clinics* subscription prices. All prices are subject to change without notice. **POSTMASTER:** Send address changes to *Interventional Cardiology Clinics*, Elsevier Health Sciences Division, Subscription Customer Service, 3251 Riverport Lane, Maryland Heights, MO 63043. **Customer Service: Telephone: 1-800-654-2452** (U.S. and Canada); **1-314-447-8871** (outside U.S. and Canada). **Fax: 1-314-447-8029. E-mail: journalscustomerservice-usa@elsevier.com (for print support); journalsonlinesupport-usa@elsevier.com (for online support).**

Reprints. For copies of 100 or more of articles in this publication, please contact the Commercial Reprints Department, Elsevier Inc., 360 Park Avenue South, New York, NY 10010-1710. Tel.: 212-633-3874; Fax: 212-633-3820; E-mail: reprints@elsevier.com.

CONTRIBUTORS

EDITOR-IN-CHIEF

MATTHEW J. PRICE, MD
Director, Cardiac Catheterization Laboratory,
Division of Cardiovascular Diseases, Scripps
Clinic, Assistant Professor, Scripps
Translational Science Institute, La Jolla,
California

EDITOR

EHRIN J. ARMSTRONG, MD, MSc
Associate Professor of Medicine, Section of
Cardiology, Denver VA Medical Center,
University of Colorado School of Medicine,
Denver, Colorado

AUTHORS

VIKAS AGGARWAL, MD, MPH
Assistant Professor of Medicine; Division of
Cardiology, Department of Internal Medicine,
Section of Interventional Cardiology, Lewis
Katz School of Medicine, Temple University,
Philadelphia, Pennsylvania

EHRIN J. ARMSTRONG, MD, MSc
Associate Professor of Medicine, Section of
Cardiology, Denver VA Medical Center,
University of Colorado School of Medicine,
Denver, Colorado

HERBERT D. ARONOW, MD, MPH, FACC,
FSCAI, FSVM
Cardiovascular Institute, Warren Alpert
Medical School of Brown University,
Providence, Rhode Island

SUBHASH BANERJEE, MD
Division of Cardiology, Department of
Medicine, University of Texas Southwestern
Medical Center, Veterans Affairs North Texas
Health Care System, Dallas, Texas

MATTHEW C. BUNTE, MD, MS
Assistant Professor of Medicine, Saint Luke's
Mid America Heart Institute, St Luke's
Hospital, University of Missouri-Kansas City
School of Medicine, Kansas City, Missouri

PRATIK K. DALAL, MD
Department of Cardiovascular Diseases,
University of Texas Health Science Center,
San Antonio, Texas

BARBARA A. DANEK, MD
Division of Cardiology, Department of
Medicine, Veterans Affairs North Texas Health
Care System, Dallas, Texas

JAY GIRI, MD, MPH
Assistant Professor of Medicine,
Cardiovascular Medicine Division, Perelman
Center, Hospital of the University of
Pennsylvania; Penn Cardiovascular Quality,
Outcomes, and Evaluative Research Center,
University of Pennsylvania, Philadelphia,
Pennsylvania

STEPHAN HEO, MD
Cardiovascular Institute, Warren Alpert
Medical School of Brown University,
Providence, Rhode Island

HAEKYUNG JEON-SLAUGHTER, PhD
Division of Cardiology, Department of
Medicine, University of Texas Southwestern
Medical Center, Veterans Affairs North Texas
Health Care System, Dallas, Texas

HOUMAN KHALILI, MD
Division of Cardiology, Department of
Medicine, University of Texas Southwestern
Medical Center, Veterans Affairs North Texas
Health Care System, Dallas, Texas

TAISEI KOBAYASHI, MD
Interventional Cardiology Fellow,
Cardiovascular Medicine Division, Perelman
Center, Hospital of the University of
Pennsylvania; Penn Cardiovascular Quality,
Outcomes, and Evaluative Research Center,
University of Pennsylvania, Philadelphia,
Pennsylvania

DAMIANOS G. KOKKINIDIS, MD
Postdoctoral Fellow, Section of Cardiology,
Denver VA Medical Center, University of
Colorado School of Medicine, Denver,
Colorado

ANANYA KONDAPALLI, MD
Division of Cardiology, Department of
Medicine, University of Texas Southwestern
Medical Center, Dallas, Texas

VLADIMIR LAKHTER, DO
Cardiology Fellow; Division of Cardiology,
Department of Internal Medicine, Section of
Interventional Cardiology, Lewis Katz School
of Medicine, Temple University, Philadelphia,
Pennsylvania

JUN LI, MD
Division of Cardiovascular Medicine,
Department of Interventional Cardiology,
Harrington Heart and Vascular Institute,
University Hospitals Cleveland Medical
Center; Department of Medicine, Case
Western Reserve University School of
Medicine, Cleveland, Ohio

ASHWIN NATHAN, MD
Cardiovascular Diseases Fellow,
Cardiovascular Medicine Division, Perelman
Center, Hospital of the University of
Pennsylvania; Penn Cardiovascular Quality,
Outcomes, and Evaluative Research Center,
University of Pennsylvania, Philadelphia,
Pennsylvania

SAHIL A. PARIKH, MD, FACC, FSCAI
Director, Endovascular Services, Associate
Professor of Medicine, Division of Cardiology,
Department of Medicine, Center for
Interventional Vascular Therapy, Columbia
University Medical Center/NY Presbyterian
Hospital, Columbia University College of
Physicians and Surgeons, New York, New York

SANDEEP M. PATEL, MD
Division of Cardiovascular Medicine,
Department of Interventional Cardiology,
Harrington Heart and Vascular Institute,
University Hospitals Cleveland Medical
Center; Department of Medicine, Case
Western Reserve University School of
Medicine, Cleveland, Ohio

ANAND PRASAD, MD, FACC, FSCAI, RPVI
Department of Cardiovascular Diseases,
University of Texas Health Science Center, San
Antonio, Texas

ANDREW F. PROUSE, MD
Cardiology and Vascular Medicine Fellow,
Division of Cardiology, University of Colorado
School of Medicine, University of Colorado,
Aurora, Colorado

ROBERT K. ROGERS, MD, MSc, RPVI
Associate Professor, Program Director,
Vascular Medicine & Intervention,
Interventional Cardiology, Associate Professor
of Medicine; Division of Cardiology, University
of Colorado School of Medicine, University of
Colorado, Aurora, Colorado

**NICOLAS W. SHAMMAS, MD, EJD, MS,
FACC, FSCAI, FICA, FSVM**
Research Director, Midwest Cardiovascular
Research Foundation, Davenport, Iowa;
Adjunct Clinical Associate Professor of
Medicine, University of Iowa, Iowa City, Iowa;
Interventional Cardiologist, Genesis Heart
Institute, Cardiovascular Medicine, PC,
Davenport, Iowa

MEHDI H. SHISHEHBOR, DO, MPH, PhD
Robert and Suzanne Tomsich Department of
Cardiovascular Medicine, Cleveland Clinic,
Cleveland, Ohio

PETER SOUKAS, MD
Cardiovascular Institute, Warren Alpert
Medical School of Brown University,
Providence, Rhode Island

RAMI TZAFRIRI, PhD
Director of Research and Innovation, CBSET
Inc, Lexington, Massachusetts

JAVIER A. VALLE, MD, MSc
Interventional Cardiology Fellow, Division of
Cardiology, VA Eastern Colorado Healthcare
System, University of Colorado School of
Medicine, Denver, Colorado

STEPHEN W. WALDO, MD
Division of Cardiology, VA Eastern Colorado
Healthcare System, University of Colorado,
Denver, Colorado

CONTENTS

Preface: Endovascular Treatment of Peripheral Artery Disease and   **xi**
Critical Limb Ischemia
Ehrin J. Armstrong

Current Status and Outcomes of Iliac Artery Endovascular Intervention   **167**
Vladimir Lakhter and Vikas Aggarwal

Aortoiliac occlusive disease (AIOD) is widely prevalent and leads to significant limitations in patient quality of life. All patients with aortoiliac occlusive disease should be managed with approved medical therapies in addition to a supervised exercise program. Persistence of significant symptoms despite noninvasive therapy should prompt further management with endovascular revascularization. Although patients with the most complex cases of AIOD anatomy may ultimately require surgery, advances in endovascular techniques have made it possible to treat most of these patients with AIOD using an endovascular-first approach.

Is Common Femoral Artery Stenosis Still a Surgical Disease?   **181**
Stephan Heo, Peter Soukas, and Herbert D. Aronow

Surgical endarterectomy has long been the standard approach for treating atherosclerotic stenosis in the common femoral artery. Its major advantage is the associated long-term patency, which approaches 95% at 5 years. Nevertheless, recent studies have suggested that percutaneous treatment may be a valid alternative to surgery.

Current Endovascular Management of Acute Limb Ischemia   **189**
Javier A. Valle and Stephen W. Waldo

Acute limb ischemia is a vascular emergency, threatening the viability of the affected limb and requiring immediate recognition and treatment. Even with revascularization of the affected extremity, acute limb ischemia is associated with significant morbidity and mortality resulting in up to a 15% risk of amputation during the initial hospitalization and a 1 in 5 risk of mortality within 1 year of the index event. This review summarizes the current management of acute limb ischemia. Understanding the diagnosis and therapeutic options will aid clinicians in treating these critically ill patients.

Mechanisms Underlying Drug Delivery to Peripheral Arteries   **197**
Jun Li, Rami Tzafriri, Sandeep M. Patel, and Sahil A. Parikh

Delivery of drugs onto arterial targets via endovascular devices commands several principles: dissolution, diffusion, convection, drug binding, barriers to absorption, and interaction between the drug, delivery vehicle, and accepting arterial wall. The understanding of drug delivery in the coronary vasculature is vast; there is ongoing work needed in the peripheral arteries. There are differences that account for some failures of application of coronary technology into the peripheral vascular space. Breakthroughs in peripheral vascular interventional techniques building on current technologies require investigators willing to acknowledge the similarities and differences between these different vascular territories, while developing technologies adapted for peripheral arteries.

Drug-Coated Balloons: Current Outcomes and Future Directions   **217**
Ananya Kondapalli, Barbara A. Danek, Houman Khalili, Haekyung Jeon-Slaughter, and Subhash Banerjee

Paclitaxel-coated drug-coated balloons have significantly improved short-term and mid-term clinical outcomes in patients with symptomatic femoropopliteal peripheral artery disease. However, long-term results are awaited. Furthermore, the clinical success of drug-coated balloons in the infrapopliteal peripheral arteries has been more modest and overall similar to traditional balloon angioplasty, and remains an area of unmet clinical need. This article provides an overview of the clinical evidence for paclitaxel-coated balloons in the femoropopliteal and infrapopliteal peripheral artery distributions and future directions in this area.

Nitinol Self-Expanding Stents for the Superficial Femoral Artery   **227**
Ashwin Nathan, Taisei Kobayashi, and Jay Giri

The superficial femoral artery is a complex artery subject to a unique set of biomechanical loading conditions in its course through the leg. Plain balloon angioplasty and balloon-expandable stents had unacceptably high rates of restenosis, necessitating target vessel revascularization. Nitinol alloy is well suited to provide the strength and flexibility needed of stents to withstand the external forces posed by the environment of the superficial femoral artery. Advances in stent technology with the addition of a slow-releasing antiproliferative agent and changes in scaffold design have shown promise in reducing the rates of stent fracture and in-stent restenosis.

Current Role of Atherectomy for Treatment of Femoropopliteal and Infrapopliteal Disease   **235**
Nicolas W. Shammas

Atherectomy improves the acute procedural success of a procedure whether treating de novo or restenotic (including in-stent) disease. Intermediate follow-up results seem to be in favor of atherectomy in delaying and reducing the need for repeat revascularization in patients with femoropopliteal in-stent restenosis. Recent data suggest that avoiding cutting into the external elastic lamina is an important factor in reducing restenosis. The interplay between directional atherectomy and drug-coated balloons is unclear.

Contemporary Outcomes of Endovascular Intervention for Critical Limb Ischemia   **251**
Pratik K. Dalal and Anand Prasad

Critical limb ischemia (CLI) remains a significant cause of morbidity and mortality in patients with peripheral arterial disease. Optimal treatment strategies for CLI remain controversial. The only randomized trial comparing surgical with endovascular revascularization suggests no significant difference in limb salvage between open surgical bypass and angioplasty. Although novel endovascular strategies are now available, their efficacies remain largely untested in a randomized fashion. This review provides an overview of the data surrounding contemporary outcomes of endovascular therapy with an emphasis on current knowledge gaps.

Inframalleolar Intervention for Limb Preservation   **261**
Javier A. Valle, Andrew F. Prouse, and Robert K. Rogers

Critical limb ischemia (CLI) is a relatively prevalent and highly morbid condition. Patients with CLI have a poor prognosis, especially in the setting of incomplete revascularization. Traditionally, achieving optimal revascularization has been limited by the high prevalence of small-vessel disease in this population. More recently, advanced endovascular techniques, increased operator experience, and new technologies have enabled complete revascularization of inframalleolar disease with encouraging clinical results. In this article, we present an approach to endovascular therapy for inframalleolar revascularization of patients with CLI.

Angiosome-Guided Intervention in Critical Limb Ischemia   **271**
Matthew C. Bunte and Mehdi H. Shishehbor

The goals of treatment for critical limb ischemia (CLI) are alleviation of ischemic rest pain, healing of arterial insufficiency ulcers, and improving quality of life, thereby preventing limb loss and CLI-related mortality. Arterial revascularization is the foundation of a contemporary approach to promote amputation-free survival. Angiosome-directed revascularization has become a popular theory of reperfusion, whereby anatomically directed arterial flow is restored straight to the wound bed. Innovations in endovascular revascularization combined with a multidisciplinary strategy of wound care accelerate progress in CLI management. This article highlights advances in CLI management, including the clinical relevance of angiosome-directed revascularization, and provides considerations for future treatment of CLI.

Emerging and Future Therapeutic Options for Femoropopliteal and   **279**
Infrapopliteal Endovascular Intervention
Damianos G. Kokkinidis and Ehrin J. Armstrong

Despite recent advances in endovascular therapy for peripheral artery disease, current technologies remain limited by rates of long-term restenosis and application to complex lesion subsets. This article presents data on upcoming therapies, including novel drug-coated balloons, drug-eluting stents, bioresorbable scaffolds, novel drug delivery therapies to target arteries, techniques to limit postangioplasty dissection, and treatment of severely calcified lesions.

ENDOVASCULAR TREATMENT OF PERIPHERAL ARTERY DISEASE AND CRITICAL LIMB ISCHEMIA

FORTHCOMING ISSUES

July 2017
Interventional Heart Failure
Srihari S. Naidu, *Editor*

October 2017
Transcatheter Closure of Patent Foramen Ovale
Matthew J. Price, *Editor*

RECENT ISSUES

January 2017
Antiplatelet and Anticoagulation Therapy in PCI
Dominick J. Angiolillo and Matthew J. Price, *Editors*

October 2016
Controversies in the Management of STEMI
Timothy D. Henry, *Editor*

ISSUE OF RELATED INTEREST

Cardiology Clinics, February 2015 (Vol. 33, No. 1)
Vascular Disease
Leonardo C. Clavijo, *Editor*
Available at: http://www.cardiology.theclinics.com/

THE CLINICS ARE NOW AVAILABLE ONLINE!

Access your subscription at:
www.theclinics.com

PREFACE

Endovascular Treatment of Peripheral Artery Disease and Critical Limb Ischemia

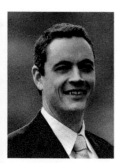

Ehrin J. Armstrong, MD
Editor

Peripheral artery disease is a common but frequently underrecognized cause of major morbidity and mortality. Increasingly, patients with symptomatic peripheral artery disease are treated with endovascular therapies, rather than more invasive surgical approaches. With the rapid development of techniques and new tools, there is a strong need for expert consensus, education, and outcomes research in peripheral artery disease. This issue provides a comprehensive and contemporary overview of the endovascular management of peripheral artery disease, with a focus on both technical aspects of intervention and clinical outcomes from recent clinical registries and trials.

The first three articles in this issue of *Interventional Cardiology Clinics* discuss emerging areas of outcomes-based evidence in the treatment of aortoiliac lesions (Current Status and Outcomes of Iliac Artery Endovascular Intervention), common femoral artery disease (Is Common Femoral Artery Stenosis Still a Surgical Disease?), and acute limb ischemia (Current Endovascular Management of Acute Limb Ischemia).

The next set of articles present emerging evidence for novel technologies to treat advanced peripheral artery disease, including anti-restenotic drug delivery (Mechanisms Underlying Drug Delivery to Peripheral Arteries), drug-coated balloons (Drug-Coated Balloons: Current Outcomes and Future Directions), new stent technologies (New Generation Nitinol and Drug-Eluting Stents for Treatment of Femoropopliteal Peripheral Artery Disease), and atherectomy devices (Current Role of Atherectomy for Treatment of Femoropopliteal and Infrapopliteal Disease).

Finally, this issue concludes with articles focused on novel therapeutic approaches for patients with critical limb ischemia. These articles include recent outcomes (Contemporary Outcomes of Endovascular Intervention for Critical Limb Ischemia), novel techniques (Inframalleolar Intervention and Extreme Access for Limb Preservation), new approaches (Angiosome-Guided Intervention in Critical Limb Ischemia), and new devices (Emerging and Future Therapeutic Options for Femoropopliteal and Infrapopliteal Endovascular Intervention).

On behalf of the authors, I hope that these articles provide state-of-the-art technical and clinical data that will ultimately improve the outcomes of our patients with peripheral artery disease.

Ehrin J. Armstrong, MD
Section of Cardiology
Denver VA Medical Center
University of Colorado School of Medicine
1055 Clermont Street
Denver, CO 80220, USA
E-mail address:
Ehrin.armstrong@gmail.com

Intervent Cardiol Clin 6 (2017) xi
http://dx.doi.org/10.1016/j.iccl.2017.01.001
2211-7458/17/© 2017 Published by Elsevier Inc.

PREFACE

Current Status and Outcomes of Iliac Artery Endovascular Intervention

Vladimir Lakhter, DO, Vikas Aggarwal, MD, MPH*

KEYWORDS

• Iliac artery intervention • Endovascular intervention • Iliac stent • Peripheral artery disease

KEY POINTS

• Work-up of patients with suspected aortoiliac occlusive disease (AIOD) requires a comprehensive approach using physical examination and multimodality imaging.
• Initial approach to the management of symptoms in patients with AIOD should include medical and exercise therapy.
• Iliac artery interventions have a high rate of technical success and excellent long-term patency.

INTRODUCTION

Lower extremity peripheral artery disease (PAD) is common and affects up to 8 million to 12 million Americans.[1] Occlusive disease of the infrarenal aorta and iliac arteries (aortoiliac occlusive disease [AIOD]) represented up to half of all patients with lower extremity PAD in a large series.[2] In the past, aortoiliac disease has been largely managed with surgical bypass grafting, but recent advances in endovascular techniques now allow percutaneous revascularization in most patients with AIOD regardless of disease complexity. This so-called endovascular-first approach is largely becoming standard of care at most institutions worldwide. This article provides a comprehensive review of AIOD endovascular revascularization strategies and outcomes.

ANATOMY

The distal abdominal aorta divides into the right and left common iliac arteries (CIAs), with each iliac artery typically measuring approximately 8 to 10 mm in diameter. The CIA subsequently bifurcates into the internal iliac artery (IIA) and the external iliac artery (EIA), each of which has a diameter of, on average, 6 to 8 mm. The EIA continues its downward course and becomes the common femoral artery (CFA) after crossing the inguinal ligament. The inferior epigastric artery arises from the CFA at the level of the inguinal ligament and delineates an important angiographic landmark above which CFA access should not be attempted. The inferior boundary for CFA access is the bifurcation of the CFA into the profunda femoris and superficial femoral artery (SFA).

The anatomic complexity of AIOD is commonly classified according to the 2007 Inter-Society Consensus for the Management of Peripheral Arterial Disease (Transatlantic Intersociety Consensus [TASC] II) guidelines.[3] TASC II guidelines stratify AIOD into 4 lesion types of increasing complexity (A–D) (Fig. 1). Type A lesions represent unilateral/bilateral CIA stenosis or short (≤3 cm) unilateral/bilateral EIA stenosis. Type B lesions include short (≤3 cm) infrarenal aortic stenosis, unilateral CIA occlusion, EIA occlusion proximal to the origin of the CFA, and single or multiple EIA stenosis

Disclosure: The authors have nothing to disclose.
Division of Cardiology, Department of Internal Medicine, Section of Interventional Cardiology, Lewis Katz School of Medicine, Temple University, 3401 North Broad Street, C945, Philadelphia, PA 19140, USA
* Corresponding author.
E-mail address: vikas.aggarwal@tuhs.temple.edu

Type A lesions

- Unilateral or bilateral stenoses of CIA
- Unilateral or bilateral single short (≤3 cm) stenosis of EIA

Type B lesions:

- Short (≤3 cm) stenosis of infrarenal aorta
- Unilateral CIA occlusion
- Single or multiple stenosis totaling 3–10 cm involving the EIA not extending into the CFA
- Unilateral EIA occlusion not involving the origins of internal iliac or CFA

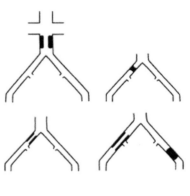

Type C lesions

- Bilateral CIA occlusions
- Bilateral EIA stenoses 3–10 cm long not extending into the CFA
- Unilateral EIA stenosis extending into the CFA
- Unilateral EIA occlusion that involves the origins of internal iliac and/or CFA
- Heavily calcified unilateral EIA occlusion with or without involvement of origins of internal iliac and/or CFA

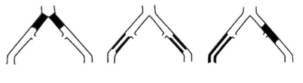

Type D lesions

- Infra-renal aortoiliac occlusion
- Diffuse disease involving the aorta and both iliac arteries requiring treatment
- Diffuse multiple stenoses involving the unilateral CIA, EIA, and CFA
- Unilateral occlusions of both CIA and EIA
- Bilateral occlusions of EIA
- Iliac stenoses in patients with AAA requiring treatment and not amenable to endograft placement or other lesions requiring open aortic or iliac surgery

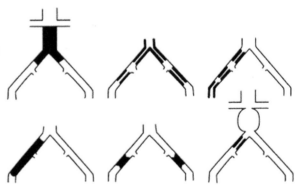

Fig. 1. TASC II AIOD lesion classification. (*Adapted from* Norgren L, Hiatt WR, Dormandy JA, et al. Inter-society consensus for the management of peripheral arterial disease (TASC II). Eur J Vasc Endovasc Surg 2007;33 Suppl 1:S52; with permission.)

3 to 10 cm in length. Type C lesions describe bilateral CIA occlusions, bilateral EIA stenosis 3 to 10 cm in length, unilateral EIA stenosis with extension into CFA, unilateral EIA occlusion involving the origin of IIA and/or CFA, and a heavily calcified unilateral EIA occlusion with or without involvement of the IIA and/or CFA. In addition, the most complex disease is described by type D lesions: infrarenal aortoiliac occlusion; diffuse infrarenal aortic stenosis involving bilateral CIAs; diffuse unilateral disease involving the CIA, EIA, and CFA; unilateral occlusion of CIA and EIA; bilateral EIA occlusions; and iliac stenoses in patients with abdominal aortic aneurysms. In the past, endovascular therapy was considered standard of care for patients with TASC A and B lesions, whereas surgical revascularization was considered to be the first-line therapy for type C and D lesions, but more recently an endovascular-first approach has

become the dominant first therapeutic option in most patients regardless of their TASC lesion type. Operator experience and expertise also play an important role in therapy choice selection.

PATHOLOGY

Specific risk factors associated with development of AIOD include traditional cardiovascular risk factors such as smoking, male gender, age, diabetes, and hyperlipidemia.[4] Patients with AIOD classically experience thigh or buttock claudication but can also present with calf claudication and atypical symptoms such as back or hip pain.[4] Involvement of the IIA, which provides blood supply to the erectile tissue of the penis via the internal pudendal artery, can result in erectile dysfunction in male patients. As a result of extensive collateral circulation, patients with AIOD are unlikely to develop limb-threatening ischemia even in the setting of complete proximal vessel occlusion. Collateral blood supply, which can arise from either the systemic (lumbar/intercostal/deep circumflex iliac/internal thoracic/inferior epigastric/obturator arteries) or visceral (celiac/superior mesenteric/inferior mesenteric arteries) circulation, usually provides enough perfusion to the distal lower extremity to result in significant attenuation of the overall ischemic burden.[5]

DIAGNOSTIC EVALUATION

Initial evaluation of patients presenting with symptoms of AIOD begins with physical examination. Either a reduction in the impulse or complete absence of the CFA pulse can be the first clue to an upstream arterial obstruction. Other physical examination findings may include weak distal pulses, lower extremity hair loss, shiny skin, or typical arterial ulceration involving the medial malleolus or the interdigital space.[6] The next step in the evaluation of symptomatic patients involves measurement of the ankle brachial index (ABI). ABI values less than 0.9 are abnormal and indicate the presence of PAD. Because the resting ABI values can be normal in patients with extensive collateral blood flow, exercise ABIs may be necessary to identify a significant exertional reduction (>10 mm Hg) in the ankle pressure. Segmental limb pressure measurements (high thigh, low thigh, upper calf, and ankle) should be performed at the time of ABI testing in order to localize the level of arterial stenosis. Normal high thigh pressure/brachial pressure index

(thigh brachial index [TBI]) is 1.1, and a TBI value less than 0.9 is suggestive of AIOD.[7] Measurement of pulse volume recordings (PVRs) can provide further information about the anatomic level of arterial obstruction. PVR tracings are obtained by filling a pneumatic cuff with enough air to occlude the venous flow at a given anatomic level. The remaining arterial impulse produces volume changes within the artery, which are picked up by the cuff and transformed into a recordable waveform. Arterial stenosis produces predictable attenuation of the waveform recording and therefore provides information regarding disease severity at that arterial segment.[7] Arterial duplex is another important diagnostic tool that can be used to assess the aortoiliac circulation. A meta-analysis of 16 studies revealed that duplex ultrasonography has a pooled sensitivity of 86% and specificity of 97% for detecting greater than or equal to 50% stenosis or an occlusion within the aortoiliac tract.[8] However, the diagnostic accuracy of this modality is significantly limited by the overlying soft tissue and bowel gas.

Diagnostic evaluation using either computed tomography angiography (CTA) or magnetic resonance angiography (MRA) could also be helpful in identifying AIOD and for providing an insight into subsequent treatment strategies such preprocedural roadmap before endovascular intervention and proximal or distal bypass graft targets. The use of multidetector CT (MDCT) technology has allowed faster acquisition of angiographic data compared with single-detector scanners. As such, MDCT has the capability of imaging the infrarenal aorta and the entire distal arterial supply of the lower extremity with a single bolus of contrast.[9] Following angiographic acquisition, postprocessing tools such as Terarecon (Foster City, CA) can be used for multiplanar reconstruction of the raw data set, which is useful for preprocedural planning. In a meta-analysis of 10 studies evaluating the use of CTA in evaluation of PAD, Sun and colleagues[10] reported a high sensitivity (92%), specificity (94%), and accuracy (93%) of CTA for detecting AIOD compared with digital subtraction angiography. The main limitation of CTA is the presence of heavy calcification, which is more prevalent in patients with diabetes and/or end-stage renal disease.[11] In these patients, arterial wall calcification significantly impairs image interpretation.[12] Unlike CTA, gadolinium-enhanced MRA is not subject to the same imaging limitations in the setting of arterial calcification.[11] Compared with conventional angiography, MRA has a pooled sensitivity of 97.5% and specificity of 96.2%.[13] Nevertheless, this imaging modality may not be a good option for patients with renal insufficiency (because of concern for nephrogenic systemic sclerosis), implanted pacemakers, hip prosthesis, or prior arterial stenting.

Contrast angiography using digital subtraction serves as the gold standard imaging modality in the work-up of AIOD. Aortoiliac stenosis involving more than 75% of the luminal diameter is considered hemodynamically significant. In the case of an intermediate stenosis (50%–75%) and stenoses of uncertain severity, translesional pressure gradient assessment is recommended. A pressure gradient of greater than 10 mm Hg or a peak postvasodilatory gradient of 10 to 15 mm Hg is considered hemodynamically significant.[4,14]

MEDICAL THERAPY

Medical therapy for all lower extremity PAD (including AIOD) should always be optimized first to minimize patients' symptoms as well as to reduce the risk of subsequent cardiovascular and limb events. All patients with PAD should be prescribed 1 or more antiplatelet agents such as aspirin, clopidogrel, prasugrel, or ticagrelor. In a meta-analysis of randomized trials evaluating the use of aspirin in patients with PAD, Berger and colleagues[15] found a significant reduction in the incidence of nonfatal stroke (relative risk [RR], 0.66; 95% confidence interval [CI], 0.47–0.94) and a nonsignificant reduction in the rate of major adverse cardiovascular events, defined as nonfatal myocardial infarction, nonfatal stroke, and cardiovascular death (RR, 0.88; 95% CI, 0.76–1.04), in the aspirin group compared with placebo. The current American College of Cardiology (ACC)/American Heart Association (AHA) guidelines recommend daily aspirin at a dose of 75 mg to 325 mg for prevention of cardiovascular death, myocardial infarction, and stroke in all patients with PAD.[16] Based on the results of the CAPRIE (Clopidogrel versus aspirin in patients at risk of ischaemic events) trial, which showed superior efficacy of clopidogrel compared with aspirin in reducing the rates of major adverse cardiovascular events in patients with PAD, current guidelines suggest clopidogrel 75 mg daily as an alternative to aspirin.[17] The combination of aspirin and clopidogrel may be reasonable in patients with PAD at the highest risk of adverse cardiac events; however, this approach increases the risk of bleeding.[18] Current guidelines also recommend using cilostazol (class 1 recommendation) to alleviate symptoms and increase the walking distance in patients with PAD experiencing intermittent claudication.[19] Pentoxifylline is recommended as an alternative to cilostazol (class IIb).

Another important noninvasive therapy in managing patients with PAD and claudication is supervised exercise. The CLEVER (Claudication: Exercise Versus Endoluminal Revascularization) study (supervised exercise versus primary stenting for claudication resulting from aortoiliac peripheral artery disease) randomized 111 patients with aortoiliac disease to optimal medical therapy, optimal medical therapy plus supervised exercise, or optimal medical therapy plus stenting.[20] Peak walking time increased the most in the supervised exercise group compared with the other groups. In comparison, scores from quality-of-life questionnaires were highest in the stenting group. The results of this study establish supervised exercise as an important therapeutic modality for all patients with PAD (including those with AIOD).

INDICATIONS FOR INVASIVE INTERVENTION

The 2014 SCAI consensus statement outlines specific clinical scenarios under which intervention for AIOD should be considered.[21] Intervention for AIOD is considered appropriate in the setting of (1) greater than or equal to 50% stenosis (or a stenosis with a mean translesional gradient >5 mm Hg) of the distal abdominal aorta or CIA in patients who experience moderate claudication or major tissue loss despite optimal medical and supervised exercise therapy; (2) greater than or equal to 50% stenosis (or a stenosis with a mean translesional gradient >5 mm Hg) of the IIA or EIA in patients with moderate to severe buttock, hip, or calf claudication or major tissue loss despite optimal medical and supervised exercise therapy; and (3) significant aortoiliac stenosis in asymptomatic patients who require vascular access for other therapies (ie, mechanical circulatory support, transcatheter cardiac valvular therapies). Intervention may also be appropriate in the setting of (1) AIOD and greater than or equal to 50% stenosis in patients with lifestyle-limiting claudication who have not failed medical/exercise therapy but in whom the risk/benefit ratio favors intervention; and (2) in patients with an IIA stenosis greater than or equal to 50% in severity who experience vasculogenic erectile dysfunction.

Overall, medical therapy and a supervised exercise program should be prescribed to all patients with PAD. Those patients who continue to have life-limiting symptoms or tissue loss despite noninvasive therapy should then be referred for revascularization.

TECHNICAL ASPECTS
Access
Identifying the appropriate anatomic site for vascular access is the first, and often the most important, decision for the operator. Common options for arterial access include ipsilateral retrograde CFA, contralateral antegrade CFA, and brachial artery access. The main determinant guiding the selection of arterial access is lesion anatomy and location of proximal and distal stumps in chronic total occlusions (CTOs).

Diagnostic Angiography
Digital subtraction angiography (DSA) is the standard approach to imaging of the aortoiliac circulation. Contralateral CFA access or left radial or brachial access approaches often allow ideal visualization of aortoiliac anatomy and disease. Diagnostic angiography using digital subtraction can often be performed using a nonselective abdominal aortic injection or a selective angiogram using a crossover catheter, such as a Rim (AngioDynamics), Cobra (Angio-Dynamics), or Simmons (Terumo). The Omni-Flush (AngioDynamics) pigtail catheter allows for both a nonselective pigtail-like injection in the abdominal aorta as well as selective engagement of the contralateral common iliac. The subsequent access strategy for intervention is then governed by lesion location and anatomy, as described later. In order to reduce motion artifact, patients should be asked to hold their breath during DSA of the infrarenal aorta and the iliac runoff. Given the significant tortuosity of the iliac vessels, contralateral oblique angulation (30°) should be used to visualize the origin of the EIA and CIA bifurcation. Ipsilateral oblique angulation (30°) is used to visualize the CFA bifurcation.

Interventional Technique
Ipsilateral retrograde CFA access allows a straight and direct transmission of force across an arterial stenosis and is therefore the access of choice in situations in which it is feasible. However, effective delivery of force across a lesion is only possible if there is enough distance between the stenosis and arteriotomy site. Therefore, ipsilateral access can be successfully used in the setting of CIA or proximal EIA stenosis.

If a CIA occlusion is present, the ipsilateral approach can still be performed as long as the vessel reconstitutes via collateral flow at the level of the proximal EIA. The ipsilateral retrograde approach is often challenging if the vessel reconstitutes below the level of proximal EIA, because there may not be enough distance between the access site and stenosis to generate enough force to cross the lesion.

Contralateral up-and-over (antegrade) access is generally used in the management of isolated EIA stenosis/occlusions (Figs. 2 and 3) and distal CIA lesions that extend into the mid-EIA to distal EIA. This approach allows revascularization of a stenosis that is anatomically too close to an ipsilateral arteriotomy site. Successful engagement and subsequent lesion crossing from the contralateral access approach depends largely on the presence of adequate stump length within the contralateral CIA. This approach allows selective engagement of the common iliac ostium from the contralateral access. Subsequently, a curved-tip braided sheath, such as a 45-cm Ansel 2 (Cook) or Flexor Raabe (Cook) guiding sheath, can be used up and over for the intervention. Long braided sheaths allow a more effective transmission of force across an arterial stenosis.

A regular brite tip sheath is otherwise sufficient when approaching these lesions from an ipsilateral retrograde approach. Another important consideration is the introducer sheath size. Given the increased risk of perforations with CTOs, the authors recommend using a 7-Fr sheath system. This system allows for seamless covered stent placement if needed.

Brachial artery access is generally reserved for management of CIA occlusions involving the proximal or ostial CIA, which cannot be approached from the contralateral or ipsilateral CFA because of inadequate stump length (such as a flush CIA occlusion extending into the mid-EIA or distal EIA). Fig. 4 shows the suggested access strategies with different lesion anatomies. Left brachial artery access is preferred to right brachial access given the shorter distance to the descending aorta and avoidance of crossing the arch vessels.

Crossing Technique
Our initial approach to crossing an arterial stenosis or an occlusion is to use the 0.89-mm (0.035″) hydrophilic-coated Glidewire (Terumo)[22] supported by an 0.89-mm angled or straight glide (Terumo) support catheter. The role of the support catheter is to prevent the wire from buckling against the cap of a dense stenosis and in turn allowing for directed transmission of force.

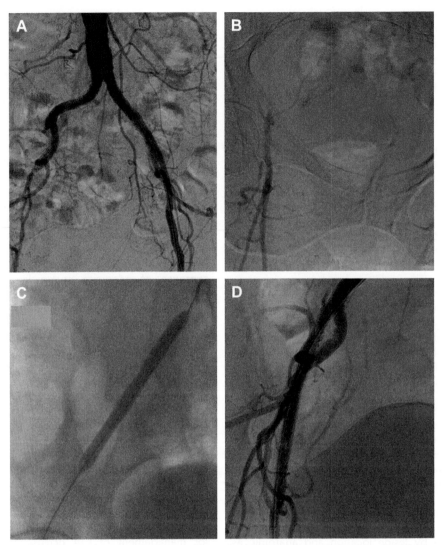

Fig. 2. Successful endovascular revascularization of a proximal EIA occlusion using a contralateral antegrade CFA approach. (*A*) Occluded proximal EIA. (*B*) Vessel reconstitution at the level of distal EIA. (*C*) Self-expanding stent placement followed by balloon post-dilation. (*D*) Restoration of blood flow within EIA following ipsilateral retrograde endovascular revascularization.

If the operator is unable to cross the stenosis/occlusion with a Glidewire/catheter support system, the authors recommend a wire-escalation strategy using a dedicated CTO crossing wire such as the Astato (Asahi) or Treasure series (Asahi) of wires. The CTO crossing wires should be used in tandem with a support catheter such as a Glide (Terumo), Quick-Cross (Spectranetics), or a CX-1 (Cook) catheter. If the lesion cannot be crossed despite the wire-escalation strategy, dedicated crossing devices such as Wildcat (Avinger), Front-Runner XP (Cordis), or a Crosser (Bard PV) catheter can be used. These catheters are designed to augment the crossing of difficult stenoses by providing adjunctive forward force using rotational spinning, blunt microdissection, or high-frequency mechanical vibration.

Wire entry into the subintimal compartment is common while attempting to cross a CTO, especially when using a hydrophilic-coated Glidewire, which follows the path of least resistance and enters the subintimal space in the setting of a dense calcified occlusion. Angiographic subintimal tracking is suspected when the wire appears to hug the margins of the vessel in a waveform fashion.[23] Under these circumstances, a dedicated reentry device, such as Pioneer

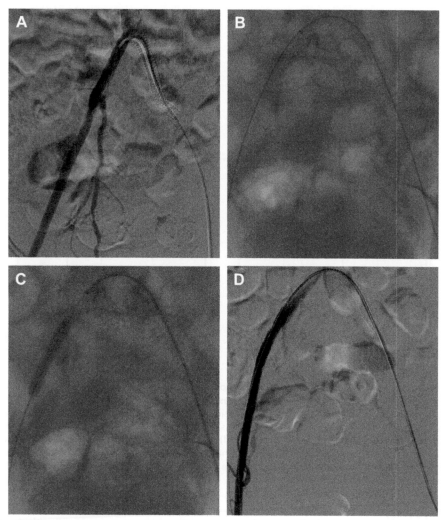

Fig. 3. Successful endovascular revascularization of a proximal EIA stenosis using a contralateral antegrade CFA approach. (*A*) Selective right lower extremity angiography showing significant proximal EIA stenosis. (*B*) Wiring across the stenosis using the contralateral retrograde approach. (*C*) Balloon expansion across the stenosis. (*D*) Significant improvement in stenosis severity after contralateral retrograde revascularization.

(Medtronic) or an Outback LTD (Cordis) catheter, can be used for reentry into the true lumen. The Pioneer catheter is an intravascular ultrasonography-based system that allows direct real-time visualization of the true lumen with its associated pulsatile color flow. The Outback LTD catheter uses angiographic guidance to reenter the true lumen using a 22-gauge nitinol reentry cannula. Ramjas and colleagues[24] described successful true lumen reentry using the Pioneer catheter in all 8 patients in whom traditional reentry techniques were unsuccessful. Furthermore, Jacobs and colleagues[25] reported successful true lumen reentry using both the Pioneer and the Outback catheters in all 24 patients undergoing endovascular treatment of iliac and SFA CTOs.

Angioplasty Technique

Following successful crossing of the arterial stenosis using a crossing catheter, the crossing wire is exchanged for a stiff 0.89-mm support wire such as Hi-Torque Supracore (Abbott Vascular) or Magic Torque (Boston Scientific). Subsequent angioplasty and stent placement is performed over these supportive wires.

The authors recommend stent placement in most patients with aortoiliac disease. Percutaneous transluminal angioplasty (PTA) as the primary strategy for management of AIOD is not recommended because 43% of patients treated with balloon angioplasty alone have a residual hemodynamically significant stenosis immediately after ballooning.[26] Furthermore, a meta-analysis of 14 studies comparing PTA with stent

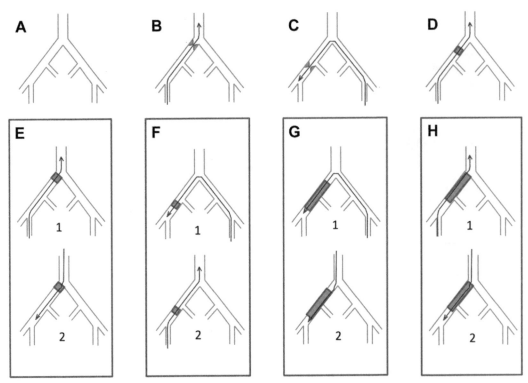

Fig. 4. (A) Normal aortoiliac anatomy; (B) crossing of a proximal CIA stenosis using ipsilateral retrograde access; (C) crossing an EIA stenosis using contralateral CFA access; (D) crossing CIA occlusion using ipsilateral retrograde access; (E, 1) preferred crossing of an ostial CIA occlusion using ipsilateral retrograde access; (E, 2) alternative crossing using left brachial access; (F, 1) preferred crossing of an EIA occlusion using contralateral CFA access; (F, 2) alternative crossing using ipsilateral access; (G, 1) preferred crossing of a long CIA occlusion extending into the EIA using contralateral CFA access; (G, 2) alternative crossing using left brachial access; (H, 1) preferred crossing of a long ostial CIA occlusion extending into the EIA using ipsilateral retrograde CFA access; (H, 2) alternative crossing using a left brachial access.

placement found stenting to have increased long-term patency rates with similar complications rates compared with PTA alone.[27]

An operator can predilate or direct the stent in most cases. Balloon predilation is particularly helpful in the setting of significant arterial calcification. However, predilation does increase the risk of arterial embolization and vessel dissection. Direct stenting can lead to stent vessel size mismatch or stent underexpansion inside severely calcified lesions. However, Scheinert and colleagues[28] reported greater than 90% success rates with less than 1% risk of distal embolization with direct stenting in iliac artery CTOs. The authors recommend careful predilation using a deliberately undersized balloon in order to avoid arterial perforation in most cases.

Stent sizing is often guided angiographically using reference vessel diameters but intravascular ultrasonography (Volcano) can also be used in select cases. The authors recommend 1:1 sizing for both balloon-expandable and self-expanding stents. Postintervention gradients should be measured in all patients undergoing stenting, with a goal of less than 10 mm Hg residual gradient at rest or with hyperemia.

Available Stents
Balloon-expandable stents
The 3 major types of commercially available stents are balloon-expandable, self-expanding, and covered stents (Table 1).[39] Balloon-expandable stents, which are made of either stainless steel or cobalt-chromium alloy, possess a high radial force or hoop strength. As such, they are preferred for treatment of CIA lesions, which are typically calcified. Balloon-expandable stents allow precise deployment and are particularly helpful when precise proximal and distal positioning is critical. The disadvantages of using a balloon-expandable stent include a higher propensity to cause an edge dissection in calcified vessels, higher risk of perforation, and less conformability to the arterial anatomy given the lack of elasticity.

Table 1
Studies summarizing the data for the currently available iliac artery stents

Study	Stent Name	Stent Type	Number of Patients/Lesions	Target Lesion Length (mm)	Primary Patency (%)	TLR, 1 y (%)
Melodie[29]	Express LD	Balloon expandable	151 patients	32.0 ± 21.7	92.1 at 6 mo	—
			163 lesions		87.8 at 2 y	
ACTIVE[30]	Assurant	Balloon expandable	123 patients	29.4 ± 14.7	99.2 at 9 mo	—
			159 lesions			
Mobility[31]	Omnilink	Balloon expandable	123 stent	45	68	14
			121 PTA	44	61	18
Krol et al,[32] 2008	Zilver	Self-expanding	34 stent	82	66	NR
			39 PTA	65	39	
CRISP US[33]	SMART	Self-expanding	102/118 SMART stent	24.7 ± 15.6	94.7 at 12 mo	13
	Wallstent		101/114 Wallstent	24.5 ± 19.1	91.1 at 12 mo	21
Mobility[34]	Absolute Pro	Self-expanding	134 stent	70	81	13
			72 PTA	64	37	55
Luminexx[35]	Lifestar	Self-expanding	134 patients	25.7 ± 18.2	94.0	3.73 (at 9 mo)
			156 lesions			
Lammer et al,[36] 2000	Viabahn	Covered self-expanding	61 lesions	69	91 at 12 mo	—
iCARUS[37]	iCAST	Covered balloon expandable	165 patients	—	—	2.9 (at 9 mo)
COBEST[38]	V12	Covered balloon expandable	62/83 V12	—	—	2.4 V12
	BMS		63/85 BMS			15.8 BMS (TVR at 18 mo)

Abbreviations: BMS, bare metal stent; NR, not reported; TLR, target lesion revascularization.

Commonly available balloon-expandable stents include the Express LD (Boston Scientific), Assurant (Medtronic), and Omnilink (Abbott Vascular) stents. The Express LD stent's flexible stainless steel framework allows it to maintain significant radial strength and radiopacity. Assurant cobalt-chromium alloy stents are designed to have a smaller cell size, which allows superior flexibility while maintaining radial strength and radiopacity. The Omnilink stent, which is also composed of cobalt-chromium alloy, has a multilink design that results in a more flexible stent. Table 1 lists studies on various stent choices in patients with AIOD.

Self-expanding stents
Self-expanding stents are most commonly composed of nitinol (nickel-titanium alloy) and possess an outward springlike property that allows them to expand in an outward fashion on unsheathing. Although more flexible, self-expanding stents have lower hoop strength compared with balloon-expandable stents. These properties allow self-expanding stents to conform with the vessel tortuosity. Because of this property, self-expanding stents are preferred in locations (such as the EIA) where significant tortuosity is often encountered. The authors believe that these properties also decrease the risk of perforation with self-expanding stents compared with balloon-expandable stents. However, given these properties and deployment mechanism, only the proximal edge of these stents can be positioned precisely. Another challenge with self-expanding stents is their inability to dilate more than the initial size, therefore self-expanding stents should never be undersized, in order to avoid malposition.

Commonly available self-expanding stents include Zilver (Cook), SMART (Cordis), Absolute Pro (Abbott), Complete SE (Medtronic), EPIC (Boston Scientific), and Lifestar (Bard) stents. The Zilver nitinol stent has a linear cell design, which was developed to minimize stent size variability during deployment. The SMART stent is equipped with a shape-memory alloy recoverable technology in addition to 12 radiopaque markers designed to improve radiopacity. The Absolute Pro stent is made of nickel-titanium alloy, which is then premounted on a triaxial delivery system designed to increase the anatomic accuracy during stent deployment. Similar to the Absolute Pro stent, the Complete self-expanding stent was designed to have excellent accuracy during deployment as a result of a dual deployment handle and a triaxial catheter system. The EPIC stent is made of nitinol and designed to provide enhanced stent visibility during deployment. The Lifestar stent is a flexible nitinol stent that is designed to deploy in a segment-by-segment fashion. The stent's flared ends were created to reduce the possibility of stent dislocation and migration.

Covered stents
Covered stents are composed of a metallic mesh encased in polytetrafluoroethylene (PTFE) or Dacron. Presence of PTFE synthetic material prevents intimal growth over the stent surface, therefore minimizing in-stent restenosis; this helps exclude aneurysms and seal perforations when encountered. Another common indication for covered stent placement is in the treatment of in-stent restenotic lesions. Given its ability to impede intimal growth within the stent, PTFE coating can result in an increased risk of subsequent stent thrombosis.

Currently available covered stents include Viabahn (Gore) and iCAST (Atrium). The Viabahn stent is a nitinol self-expanding stent system lined with PTFE, which allows significant stent flexibility. The dual-lumen delivery catheter is used to aid in stent delivery. The iCAST stent is a balloon-expandable stainless steel stent that has an inner and an outer PTFE coating. This dual coating was developed to help facilitate an even distribution of radial stress during stent expansion.

The authors recommend using a noncovered stent in most patients and reserving a covered stent strategy for select cases with in-stent restenosis, perforations, and iliac artery aneurysms. General considerations for stent selection are described in Table 2.

Special Considerations
Ostial CIA occlusions, TASC C/D lesions, and hybrid endovascular/surgical approaches are special anatomic types that deserve extra consideration.

Ostial common iliac artery occlusion
An endovascular approach should be performed using ipsilateral retrograde access. A special consideration in the setting of an ostial CIA occlusion is the possibility of shifting the plaque during balloon inflation from the involved CIA into the opposite iliac. To prevent plaque shifting, contralateral CIA access is necessary to perform so-called kissing balloon inflation (Fig. 5). Following balloon angioplasty, simultaneous bilateral stent placement is performed with the proximal landing zone of both stents being within the lumen of the infrarenal aorta. As a result, there is an upward shift of the aortic bifurcation, which precludes any future attempts at crossover access using the contralateral CFA.

Table 2
Advantages and disadvantages of iliac artery stent types

Stent Type	Advantages	Disadvantages
Self-expanding	Highly flexible May be favored in EIA lesion	Less predictable deployment than balloon-expandable stents
Balloon expandable	Increased radial strength Predictable placement May be favored in ostial or calcified lesions	Less flexible than self-expanding stents
Covered stent	Excludes plaque/thrombus May be associated with improved patency for TASC C/D lesions	Increased risk for subsequent stent thrombosis

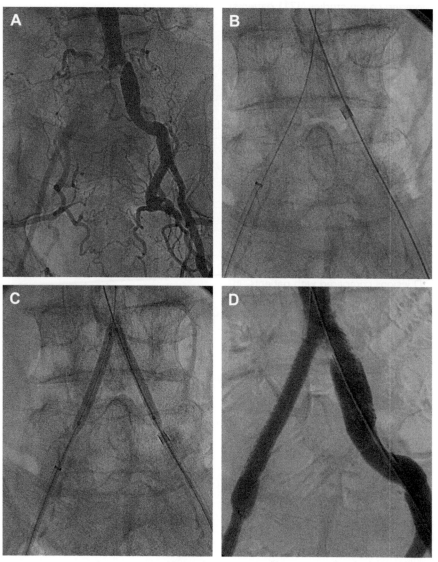

Fig. 5. (A) Occlusion of the right CIA with reconstitution at the level of distal CIA and a second lesion involving the ostium of the right CIA; (B) bilateral crossing of CIA stenoses via retrograde CFA access; (C) kissing balloon inflation; (D) successful revascularization and stenting of severe bilateral CIA disease.

Aihara and colleagues[40] evaluated the outcomes in 190 patients with AIOD who underwent bifurcation stenting using balloon-expandable or self-expanding stents. The primary patency rates were 87% at 1 year and 73% at 5 years, with an associated overall complication rate of 6.3%. The investigators did not find any differences in patency rates according to the balloon-expandable stent type.

Transatlantic Intersociety Consensus C/D lesions

Although the 2007 TASC II document recommends surgical therapy for patients with complex AIOD, endovascular intervention for TASC C and D lesions is often feasible. A systematic review of 19 nonrandomized cohort studies (1711 patients) evaluated the role of endovascular intervention in patients with AIOD and TASC C and D lesions.[41] Despite significant clinical heterogeneity between the studies, the overall results were encouraging. Most patients experienced clinical improvement of symptoms and maintained primary patency 60% to 86% of the time at 4-year or 5-year follow-up. The secondary patency rates following reintervention were 80% to 98% during the same follow-up period and were similar to those of surgical repair. Complication rates varied significantly between the studies (3%–45%). More recent data evaluating endovascular management of patients with type D lesions showed a 91.6% success rate, 77.9% 5-year primary patency rate, and a 30.5% major adverse cardiovascular and limb event rate.[42] The primary patency rate was significantly lower in patients with TASC D lesions compared with patients undergoing endovascular treatment of TASC A to C lesions.

Hybrid approach

In patients with extensive iliac disease that extends into the CFA, a hybrid approach using CFA endarterectomy in tandem with iliac stenting has been described.[43] The hybrid approach can allow treatment of longer arterial segments than is otherwise achievable with endovascular treatment alone. Chang and colleagues[44] evaluated this approach in 171 patients with extensive AIOD stenosis. The hybrid technique was successful in 98% of all patients and was associated with 60% primary and 98% secondary patency rates at 5 years.

Complications

The most common complication associated with endovascular intervention is access site–relating bleeding and hematoma formation. However, most of these cases can be managed with compressive therapy without any long-term sequelae.[45] Arterial rupture is a rare complication affecting 0.5% to 3.0% of all cases and can be managed successfully with urgent placement of a covered stent.[43] Distal embolization of plaque material is another serious complication of percutaneous revascularization. Although distal embolic protection devices can be used, no current device is approved for intervention within the aortoiliac circulation. In cases of distal embolization, either aspiration or mechanical thrombectomy can be attempted. If endovascular thrombectomy fails, surgical embolectomy may be required.[43]

SUMMARY

AIOD is widely prevalent and leads to significant limitation in patient quality of life. All patients should be managed with approved medical therapies in addition to a supervised exercise program. Persistence of significant symptoms despite noninvasive therapy should prompt further management with endovascular revascularization. Although patients with the most complex cases of AIOD may ultimately require surgery, advances in endovascular techniques have made it possible to treat most patients with AIOD using an endovascular-first approach.

REFERENCES

1. Hirsch AT, Criqui MH, Treat-Jacobson D, et al. Peripheral arterial disease detection, awareness, and treatment in primary care. JAMA 2001;286:1317–24.
2. Aboyans V, Desormais I, Lacroix P, et al. The general prognosis of patients with peripheral arterial disease differs according to the disease localization. J Am Coll Cardiol 2010;55:898–903.
3. Norgren L, Hiatt WR, Dormandy JA, et al. Inter-society consensus for the management of peripheral arterial disease (TASC II). Eur J Vasc Endovasc Surg 2007;33(Suppl 1):S1–75.
4. Neisen MJ. Endovascular management of aortoiliac occlusive disease. Semin Intervent Radiol 2009;26: 296–302.
5. Hardman RL, Lopera JE, Cardan RA, et al. Common and rare collateral pathways in aortoiliac occlusive disease: a pictorial essay. AJR Am J Roentgenol 2011;197:W519–24.
6. Spentzouris G, Labropoulos N. The evaluation of lower-extremity ulcers. Semin Intervent Radiol 2009;26:286–95.
7. Gerhard-Herman M, Gardin JM, Jaff M, et al. Guidelines for noninvasive vascular laboratory testing: a report from the American Society of Echocardiography and the Society for Vascular Medicine and Biology. Vasc Med 2006;11:183–200.

8. Koelemay MJ, den Hartog D, Prins MH, et al. Diagnosis of arterial disease of the lower extremities with duplex ultrasonography. Br J Surg 1996;83:404–9.

9. Martin ML, Tay KH, Flak B, et al. Multidetector CT angiography of the aortoiliac system and lower extremities: a prospective comparison with digital subtraction angiography. AJR Am J Roentgenol 2003;180:1085–91.

10. Sun Z. Diagnostic accuracy of multislice CT angiography in peripheral arterial disease. J Vasc Interv Radiol 2006;17:1915–21.

11. Pollak AW, Norton PT, Kramer CM. Multimodality imaging of lower extremity peripheral arterial disease: current role and future directions. Circ Cardiovasc Imaging 2012;5:797–807.

12. Ouwendijk R, Kock MC, Visser K, et al. Interobserver agreement for the interpretation of contrast-enhanced 3D MR angiography and MDCT angiography in peripheral arterial disease. AJR Am J Roentgenol 2005;185:1261–7.

13. Visser K, Hunink MG. Peripheral arterial disease: gadolinium-enhanced MR angiography versus color-guided duplex US–a meta-analysis. Radiology 2000;216:67–77.

14. Hirsch AT, Haskal ZJ, Hertzer NR, et al. ACC/AHA 2005 practice guidelines for the management of patients with peripheral arterial disease (lower extremity, renal, mesenteric, and abdominal aortic): a collaborative report from the American Association for Vascular Surgery/Society for Vascular Surgery, Society for Cardiovascular Angiography and Interventions, Society for Vascular Medicine and Biology, Society of Interventional Radiology, and the ACC/AHA Task Force on Practice Guidelines (Writing Committee to Develop Guidelines for the Management of Patients With Peripheral Arterial Disease): endorsed by the American Association of Cardiovascular and Pulmonary Rehabilitation; National Heart, Lung, and Blood Institute; Society for Vascular Nursing; TransAtlantic Inter-Society Consensus; and Vascular Disease Foundation. Circulation 2006;113:e463–654.

15. Berger JS, Krantz MJ, Kittelson JM, et al. Aspirin for the prevention of cardiovascular events in patients with peripheral artery disease: a meta-analysis of randomized trials. JAMA 2009;301:1909–19.

16. Rooke TW, Hirsch AT, Misra S, et al. 2011 ACCF/AHA focused update of the guideline for the management of patients with peripheral artery disease (updating the 2005 guideline): a report of the American College of Cardiology Foundation/American Heart Association Task Force on Practice Guidelines. J Am Coll Cardiol 2011;58:2020–45.

17. CAPRIE Steering Committee. A randomised, blinded, trial of clopidogrel versus aspirin in patients at risk of ischaemic events (CAPRIE). CAPRIE Steering Committee. Lancet 1996;348:1329–39.

18. Cacoub PP, Bhatt DL, Steg PG, et al. Patients with peripheral arterial disease in the CHARISMA trial. Eur Heart J 2009;30:192–201.

19. Anderson JL, Halperin JL, Albert NM, et al. Management of patients with peripheral artery disease (compilation of 2005 and 2011 ACCF/AHA guideline recommendations): a report of the American College of Cardiology Foundation/American Heart Association Task Force on Practice Guidelines. Circulation 2013;127:1425–43.

20. Murphy TP, Cutlip DE, Regensteiner JG, et al. Supervised exercise versus primary stenting for claudication resulting from aortoiliac peripheral artery disease: six-month outcomes from the claudication: exercise versus endoluminal revascularization (CLEVER) study. Circulation 2012;125:130–9.

21. Klein AJ, Feldman DN, Aronow HD, et al. SCAI expert consensus statement for aorto-iliac arterial intervention appropriate use. Catheter Cardiovasc Interv 2014;84:520–8.

22. Niazi K, Farooqui F, Devireddy C, et al. Comparison of hydrophilic guidewires used in endovascular procedures. J Invasive Cardiol 2009;21:397–400.

23. Sumitsuji S, Inoue K, Ochiai M, et al. Fundamental wire technique and current standard strategy of percutaneous intervention for chronic total occlusion with histopathological insights. JACC Cardiovasc Interv 2011;4:941–51.

24. Ramjas G, Thurley P, Habib S. The use of a re-entry catheter in recanalization of chronic inflow occlusions of the common iliac artery. Cardiovasc Intervent Radiol 2008;31:650–4.

25. Jacobs DL, Motaganahalli RL, Cox DE, et al. True lumen re-entry devices facilitate subintimal angioplasty and stenting of total chronic occlusions: initial report. J Vasc Surg 2006;43:1291–6.

26. Tetteroo E, van der Graaf Y, Bosch JL, et al. Randomised comparison of primary stent placement versus primary angioplasty followed by selective stent placement in patients with iliac-artery occlusive disease. Dutch Iliac Stent Trial Study Group. Lancet 1998;351:1153–9.

27. Bosch JL, Hunink MG. Meta-analysis of the results of percutaneous transluminal angioplasty and stent placement for aortoiliac occlusive disease. Radiology 1997;204:87–96.

28. Scheinert D, Schroder M, Ludwig J, et al. Stent-supported recanalization of chronic iliac artery occlusions. Am J Med 2001;110:708–15.

29. Stockx L, Poncyljusz W, Krzanowski M, et al. Express LD vascular stent in the treatment of iliac artery lesions: 24-month results from the MELODIE trial. J Endovasc Ther 2010;17:633–41.

30. Molnar RG, Gray WA. Sustained patency and clinical improvement following treatment of

atherosclerotic iliac artery disease using the Assurant cobalt iliac balloon-expandable stent system. J Endovasc Ther 2013;20:94–103.

31. Abbott Vascular [Web page]. Omnilink Elite® Vascular Balloon-Expandable Stent System. Available at: http://www.abbottvascular.com/docs/ifu/peripheral_intervention/eIFU-Omnilink-Elite.pdf. Accessed September 20, 2016.

32. Krol KL, Saxon RR, Farhat N, et al. Clinical evaluation of the Zilver vascular stent for symptomatic iliac artery disease. J Vasc Interv Radiol 2008;19:15–22.

33. Ponec D, Jaff MR, Swischuk J, et al. The Nitinol SMART stent vs Wallstent for suboptimal iliac artery angioplasty: CRISP-US trial results. J Vasc Interv Radiol 2004;15:911–8.

34. Abbott Vascular [Web page]. Absolute Pro® Vascular Self-Expanding Stent System. Available at: http://www.abbottvascular.com/docs/ifu/peripheral_intervention/eIFU_Absolute_Pro.pdf. Accessed September 22, 2016.

35. Bard Peripheral Vascular, Inc [Web page]. LifeStar™ Vascular Stent System Ordering Information. Available at: http://www.bardpv.com/wp-content/uploads/2013/07/S120118-R0-LifeStar-Vascular-Sales-Sheet.pdf. Accessed September 22, 2016.

36. Lammer J, Dake MD, Bleyn J, et al. Peripheral arterial obstruction: prospective study of treatment with a transluminally placed self-expanding stent-graft. International Trial Study Group. Radiology 2000;217:95–104.

37. Endovascular Today [Web page]. Atrium's iCast covered stent in iliac treatment supported by iCARUS study. Available at: http://evtoday.com/2012/10/atriums-icast-covered-stent-in-iliac-treatment-supported-by-icarus-study. Accessed September 22, 2016.

38. Mwipatayi BP, Thomas S, Wong J, et al. A comparison of covered vs bare expandable stents for the treatment of aortoiliac occlusive disease. J Vasc Surg 2011;54:1561–70.

39. Aggarwal V, Waldo SW, Armstrong EJ. Endovascular revascularization for aortoiliac atherosclerotic disease. Vasc Health Risk Manag 2016;12:117–27.

40. Aihara H, Soga Y, Iida O, et al. Long-term outcomes of endovascular therapy for aortoiliac bifurcation lesions in the real-AI registry. J Endovasc Ther 2014;21:25–33.

41. Jongkind V, Akkersdijk GJ, Yeung KK, et al. A systematic review of endovascular treatment of extensive aortoiliac occlusive disease. J Vasc Surg 2010;52:1376–83.

42. Suzuki K, Mizutani Y, Soga Y, et al. Efficacy and safety of endovascular therapy for aortoiliac TASC D Lesions. Angiology 2017;67(1):67–73.

43. Clair DG, Beach JM. Strategies for managing aortoiliac occlusions: access, treatment and outcomes. Expert Rev Cardiovasc Ther 2015;13:551–63.

44. Chang RW, Goodney PP, Baek JH, et al. Long-term results of combined common femoral endarterectomy and iliac stenting/stent grafting for occlusive disease. J Vasc Surg 2008;48:362–7.

45. Tsetis D, Uberoi R. Quality improvement guidelines for endovascular treatment of iliac artery occlusive disease. Cardiovasc Intervent Radiol 2008;31:238–45.

Is Common Femoral Artery Stenosis Still a Surgical Disease?

Stephan Heo, MD, Peter Soukas, MD,
Herbert D. Aronow, MD, MPH, FSCAI, FSVM*

KEYWORDS

- Common femoral artery • Atherosclerosis • Endovascular • Claudication • Critical limb ischemia
- Endarterectomy

KEY POINTS

- The morbidity of common femoral artery endarterectomy is often understated.
- Endovascular treatment for common femoral artery stenosis may be a viable treatment alternative to traditional surgical revascularization.

INTRODUCTION

The external iliac artery becomes the common femoral artery (CFA) as it passes below the inguinal ligament. The CFA is approximately 4 to 6 cm in length and 5 to 8 mm in diameter, located in the femoral triangle between the femoral vein and nerve. The CFA and its branches supply most of the thigh as well as the entirety of the leg and foot. The CFA gives rise to the largest branch of the femoral triangle, the profunda femoris, and then becomes the superficial femoral artery (SFA), which traverses along the anteromedial thigh. When atherosclerosis develops in the CFA, it can be extensive, eccentric, and heavily calcified (Fig. 1). In most patients, atherosclerosis involves the posterior wall of the CFA, whereas the anterior wall is relatively spared due to the differential wall stress along its circumference. Isolated atherosclerotic involvement of the CFA is uncommon. CFA disease can be asymptomatic, cause lifestyle-limiting claudication, and/or lead to critical limb ischemia (CLI). The CFA also may be an important site for collateral blood supply to the to the lower limb via the SFA in patients who have aorto-iliac disease and to the profunda femoris when there is SFA occlusion.

Common femoral endarterectomy with patch angioplasty had long been considered the gold standard for treating CFA disease because it was viewed as a low-risk operation requiring a small incision with excellent long-term patency rates; however, recent data suggest that morbidity after endarterectomy may be as high as 31%.[1] With evolution in technology, endovascular therapy is increasingly considered as an alternative treatment for CFA disease. Both forms of revascularization appear superior to medical therapy alone for limb-related outcomes,[2–4] but their relative safety and efficacy are less clear.

SURGICAL TREATMENT OPTIONS

Common femoral endarterectomy has been the standard approach for treating CFA stenosis for more than 60 years. Its major advantage is the associated long-term patency, which approaches 95% at 5 years. Ballotta and colleagues[5] performed an 8-year single-center prospective study of 117 patients who underwent 121 CFA endarterectomies performed under regional anesthesia. All of the arteriotomies were routinely closed with a vein patch. Postoperatively, 71% and 39% of patients

---

Disclosure Statement: None.

Cardiovascular Institute, Warren Alpert Medical School of Brown University, 593 Eddy Street, Providence, RI 02903, USA

* Corresponding author. 593 Eddy Street, RIH APC 730, Providence, RI 02903.

E-mail address: Herbert.Aronow@lifespan.org

Intervent Cardiol Clin 6 (2017) 181–187
http://dx.doi.org/10.1016/j.iccl.2016.12.002

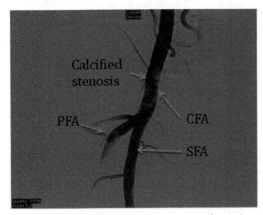

Fig. 1. Heavily calcified right CFA. PFA, profunda femoris artery.

experienced marked or moderate clinical improvement, respectively. The 5-year primary patency rate was 96% ± 3%, and the 5-year freedom from ipsilateral arterial intervention was 82% ± 7% (Fig. 2).[5,6]

Kuma and colleagues[7] also demonstrated the long-term patency of CFA endarterectomy in a retrospective examination of 118 limbs in 111 patients with claudication and CLI. The 1-year and 5-year patency for claudication and CLI were 100% and 95%, respectively.

Although CFA endarterectomy has excellent patency at 5 years, it is not a benign procedure. In a retrospective study of 1843 common femoral endarterectomies performed between 2005 and 2010 using the American College of Surgeons National Surgical Quality Improvement Program® dataset, 10% of patients returned to the operating room. Mortality and wound complications occurred in 3.4% and 8.0%, respectively. Of these, 30% and 86% occurred after hospital discharge, respectively (Fig. 3). Overall, the risk of mortality/morbidity was 15%, and more than 60% of all events occurred after discharge (Fig. 4).[8]

ENDOVASCULAR TREATMENT OPTIONS

The CFA has long been considered a suboptimal location for endovascular therapy. Heavily calcified stenosis, when present, may not respond well to balloon angioplasty, resulting in suboptimal angiographic outcomes and the need for stent placement. Balloon angioplasty also carries the risk of vessel dissection, which may require stenting. Because the CFA is located where hip flexion and extension occur, stent fracture and resultant in-stent restenosis may be more likely, resulting in poor outcomes.[9–11] In addition, stents located in the CFA may limit future surgical (ie,

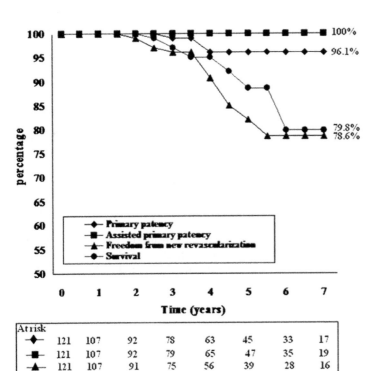

Fig. 2. Kaplan-Meier life table analysis of primary patency (diamonds), "assisted" primary patency (squares), freedom from new revascularization (triangles), and survival (circles) rates after common femoral endarterectomy. (From Ballotta E, Gruppo M, Mazzalai F, et al. Common femoral artery endarterectomy for occlusive disease: an 8 year single center prospective study. Surgery 2010;147(2):272; with permission.)

At risk								
◆	121	107	92	78	63	45	33	17
■	121	107	92	79	65	47	35	19
▲	121	107	91	75	56	39	28	16
●	117	103	87	74	53	36	26	14

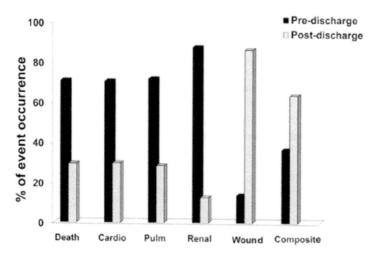

Fig. 3. Distribution of major complications before and after hospital discharge following common femoral endarterectomy. A significant percentage (30%) of deaths and cardiac and pulmonary complications occurred after hospital discharge. Most wound-related complications occurred after hospital discharge.

may prevent more proximal arterial clamping during an endarterectomy or compromise a surgical bypass anastomosis site) and endovascular (may eliminate an important location for arterial vascular access) options. Improved endovascular technology, including atherectomy devices and drug-coated balloons, may represent a potential nonstent solution for CFA disease, but there are few published data to support this approach.

Endovascular repair of the CFA may be technically challenging as well. CFA disease not infrequently involves the bifurcation. The Medina classification, a schema developed for use in coronary artery bifurcation lesions, has been applied to the CFA bifurcation as well (Fig. 5).[12] When a stent is required, a single-stent approach is most often recommended because it is simpler to execute and is associated with better outcomes.[13–15] However, when a true bifurcation lesion (Medina 1-1-1) is present,

other techniques for bifurcation reconstruction may be required (Fig. 6).[16]

Recent studies of endovascular treatment for CFA stenosis are summarized in Table 1.

New technologies and improved stent designs, such as the braided nickel-titanium alloy (Nitinol) Supera peripheral stent system (Abbott Vascular, Santa Clara, CA), are able to withstand unique stressors in the lower extremity, have shown superior stent patency and reduced stent fracture in femoropopliteal disease, and may allow for direct vessel reentry through stent struts.[19–22] Ongoing studies are assessing the safety and efficacy of this device for treatment of CFA disease.

Bioabsorbable stent implantation is also being investigated for use in the CFA. Interim analysis of a small randomized trial comparing bioabsorbable stent implantation with CFA endarterectomy found no statistically significant

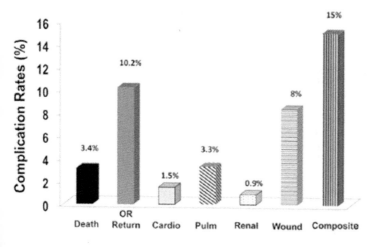

Fig. 4. Thirty-day postoperative complications after common femoral endarterectomy. Major organ dysfunction (cardiac, pulmonary, renal) was rare, but wound-related complications, operative reintervention, and mortality rates were high. OR, operating room.

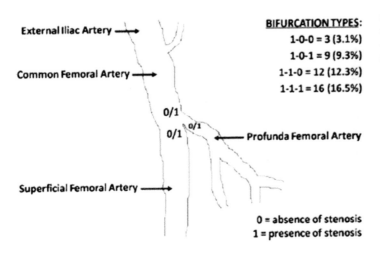

BIFURCATION TYPES:

1-0-0 = 3 (3.1%)
1-0-1 = 9 (9.3%)
1-1-0 = 12 (12.3%)
1-1-1 = 16 (16.5%)

External Iliac Artery

Common Femoral Artery

0/1

0/1

0/1

Profunda Femoral Artery

Superficial Femoral Artery

0 = absence of stenosis
1 = presence of stenosis

Fig. 5. CFA bifurcation Medina classification. 0, absence of significant stenosis; 1, presence of significant stenosis; CFA, first number; PFA, third number; SFA, second number.

difference in wound infection rates between groups (the primary endpoint); however, CFA endarterectomy was associated with more frequent complications and bioabsorbable stent implantation had poorer primary and secondary patency at 1 year (Fig. 7).[18]

Absent randomized data, many operators use balloon angioplasty (often drug-coated) with or without atherectomy, and reserve stents for flow-limiting dissection or suboptimal angiographic result. If a flow-limiting dissection does occur, a self-expanding stent as short as possible may be desired so as to allow future femoral bypass anastomosis or CFA puncture above the stent if needed. Bovini and colleagues[12] proposed an algorithm for the endovascular treatment of CFA stenosis that addresses the degree of calcification, underlying

pathophysiology (neointimal hyperplasia vs atherosclerosis), and bifurcation lesion classification (Fig. 8).

APPROPRIATE USE

In advance of release of a multispecialty Appropriate Use Criteria document on intervention for lower extremity peripheral artery disease, the Society for Cardiovascular Angiography and Interventions has published an expert consensus document on the application of endovascular intervention to patients with femoropopliteal disease (Table 2). The clinical scenarios below in Table 2 assume that lifestyle-limiting claudication has been refractory to pharmacologic therapies and a supervised exercise program.

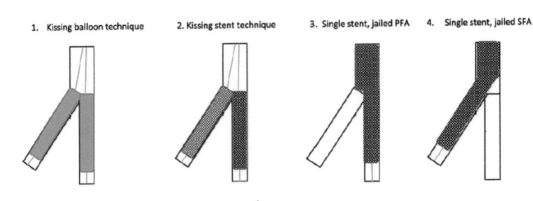

1. Kissing balloon technique   2. Kissing stent technique   3. Single stent, jailed PFA   4. Single stent, jailed SFA

PFA = Profunda femoris artery

SFA = Superficial femoral artery

Fig. 6. Techniques of reconstruction for femoral arterial bifurcation.

Table 1
Studies of endovascular treatment for common femoral artery stenosis

Author	Type of Study	Sample Size	Intervention	Results
Mehta et al,[17] 2016	Prospective observational	167	PTA alone Atherectomy plus PTA Provisional stent	Overall complications 0.6% 42.5-mo primary patency stent group 100% vs nonstented combined 77% ($P = .0424$) 20-mo atherectomy + PTA patency 92.3% vs PTA alone patency 72% ($P = .03$)
Thiney et al,[16] 2015	Prospective observational	53	Primary stenting	2-y freedom from restenosis 92.5% 2-y freedom from TLR 97% 1-y stent fracture 9%
Linni et al,[18] 2014	Randomized controlled	116	BASI vs CFE	7 site infections for CFE Postoperative stay CFE 7 d vs BASI 2 d ($P<.001$) 1-y patency CFE 100% vs BASI 84% ($P = .007$) Survival CFE 90% vs BASI 88% ($P = .51$)
Yamawaki et al,[23] 2013	Retrospective observational	104	Self-expanding stent distal CFA involving femoral bifurcation and jailed deep femoral artery	12-mo bifurcation patency 72.5% vs ostial SFA stent 52% ($P<.1$) 12-mo deep femoral artery patency Bifurcation 95.7% vs ostial SFA 100% ($P = .237$)
Bovini et al,[12] 2011	Retrospective observational	360	Balloon angioplasty 98.6% Stenting after suboptimal result 36.9%	1-y overall patency 87.5% 1-y restenosis 27.6%
Paris et al,[24] 2011	Retrospective observational	26	Balloon angioplasty Stent	30-mo claudication success 100% 30-mo CLI ABI success 70% Success of reaccess stented CFA 100%
Dattilo et al,[25] 2013	Retrospective observational	30	Balloon angioplasty	1-y survival + amp free 96% 1-y patency 88%
Stricker et al,[13] 2004	Retrospective observational	27	Balloon angioplasty Stent	30-mo patency 86% 3-y patency 83% Success reaccess stented CFA 100%
Silva et al,[14] 2004	Retrospective observational	20	Balloon angioplasty	11.4-mo event-free critical limb ischemia 90% 11.4-mo improvement in 1 Fontaine class 89%

Abbreviations: ABI, ankle-brachial pressure index; BASI, bioabsorbable stent implantation; CFA, common femoral artery; CLE, CFA endarterectomy; CLI, critical limb ischemia; PTA, percutaneous angioplasty; SFA, superficial femoral artery; TLR, target lesion revascularization.

SUMMARY

Surgery has long been viewed as the "gold standard" therapy for CFA stenosis; however, recent data have highlighted the significant incidence of wound and other complications associated with surgery. Endovascular procedures are associated with a significantly lower procedural risk compared with surgical treatment, but patency

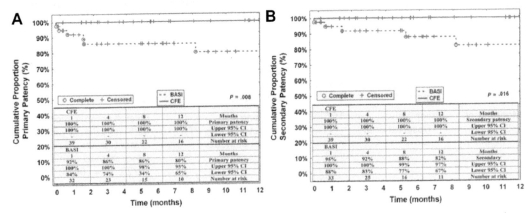

Fig. 7. Kaplan-Meier estimates of the cumulative (A) primary and (B) secondary patency rates in patients undergoing bioabsorbable stent implantation (BASI) or common femoral artery endarterectomy.

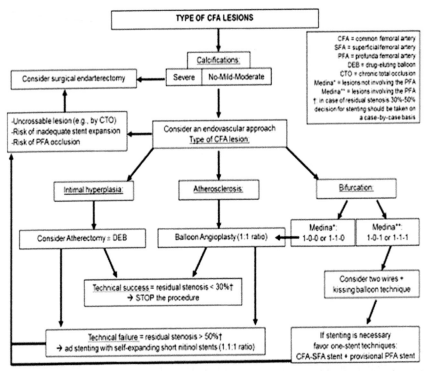

Fig. 8. Proposed treatment algorithm for CFA lesions. (*From* Bonvini RF, Rastan A, Sixt S, et al. Angioplasty and provisional stent treatment of common femoral artery lesions. J Vasc Interv Radiol 2013;24(2):180; with permission.)

Table 2 Clinical scenarios in which treatment of PAD maybe considered	
Appropriate care	CFA with >70% stenosis or CTO and the clinical need for vascular access (ie, IABP or large-bore access for TAVR or PVAD) CLI
May be appropriate care	CFA >70% or CTO with severe claudication or CLI (RC 3–6)
Rarely appropriate care	CFA >70% or CTO with mild or no symptoms (RC 0–1)

Abbreviations: CFA, common femoral artery; CLI, critical limb ischemia; CTO, chronic total occlusion; IABP, intra-aortic balloon pump; PVAD, percutaneous ventricular assist device; RC, Rutherford classification; TAVR, transcatheter aortic valve replacement.

Data from Klein A, Pinto D, Gray B, et al. SCAI expert consensus statement for femoral-popliteal arterial intervention appropriate use. Catheter Cardiovasc Interv 2014;84:529–38.

may be significantly lower than with CFA endarterectomy. Newer technologies, including atherectomy for plaque modification, drug-coated balloon angioplasty, and woven stent designs may result in improved patency but will require further study.

REFERENCES

1. Kang JL, Patel VI, Conrad MF, et al. Common femoral artery occlusive disease: contemporary results following surgical endarterectomy. J Vasc Surg 2008;48:872–7.

2. Murphy TP, Cutlip DE, Regensteiner JG, et al. Supervised exercise versus primary stenting for claudication resulting from aortoiliac peripheral artery disease: six-month outcomes from the claudication: exercise versus endoluminal revascularization (CLEVER) study. Circulation 2012;125:130–9.

3. Gardner AW, Poehlman ET. Exercise rehabilitation programs for the treatment of claudication pain. A meta-analysis. JAMA 1995;274:975–80.

4. Mays RJ, Casserly IP, Kohrt WM, et al. Assessment of functional status and quality of life in claudication. J Vasc Surg 2011;53:1410–21.

5. Ballotta E, Gruppo M, Mazzalai F, et al. Common femoral artery endarterectomy for occlusive disease: an 8 year single center prospective study. Surgery 2010;147(2):268–74.

6. Derksen WJ, Verhoeven B, van de Mortel RH, et al. Risk factors for surgical-site infection following common femoral endarterectomy. Vasc Endovascular Surg 2009;43(1):69–75.

7. Kuma S, Tanaka K, Ohmine T, et al. Clinical outcome of surgical endarterectomy for common femoral artery occlusive disease. Circ J 2016;80(4):964–9.

8. Ngyuen BN, Amdur RL, Abugideiri M, et al. Postoperative complications after common femoral endarterectomy. J Vasc Surg 2015;61(6):1489–94.

9. Norgren L, Hiatt WR, Dormandy JA, et al. Inter-society consensus for the management of peripheral arterial disease (TASC II). J Vasc Surg 2007;45:S5–67.

10. Kasapis C, Henke PK, Chetcuti SJ. Routine stent implantation vs percutaneous transluminal angioplasty in femoropopliteal artery disease: a meta-analysis of randomized controlled trials. Eur Heart J 2009;30:44–55.

11. Scheinert D, Scheinert S, Sax J. Prevalence and clinical impact of stent fractures after femoropopliteal stenting. J Am Coll Cardiol 2005;45:312–5.

12. Bovini R, Rastan A, Sixt S, et al. Endovascular treatment of common femoral artery disease, medium term outcomes of 360 procedures. J Am Coll Cardiol 2011;58(8):792–8.

13. Stricker H, Jacomella V. Stent-assisted angioplasty at the level of the common femoral artery bifurcation: midterm outcomes. J Endovasc Ther 2004;11:281–6.

14. Silva JA, White CJ, Quintana H, et al. Percutaneous revascularization for the common femoral artery for limb ischemia. Catheter Cardiovasc Interv 2004;62:230–3.

15. Zhang F, Doug L, Ge J. Simple versus complex stenting strategy for coronary artery bifurcation lesions in the drug eluting stent era; a meta analysis of randomized trials. Heart 2009;95:1676–81.

16. Thiney PO, Millon A, Boudjelit T, et al. Angioplasty of the common femoral artery and its bifurcation. Ann Vasc Surg 2015;29(5):960–7.

17. Mehta M, Zhou Y, Paty P, et al. Percutaneous common femoral artery interventions using angioplasty, atherectomy and stenting. J Vasc Surg 2016;64(2):369–79.

18. Linni K, Ugurluoglu A, Hitzl W, et al. Bioabsorbable stent implantation vs common femoral endarterectomy: early results of a randomized trial. J Endovasc Ther 2014;21:493–502.

19. Bishu K, Armstrong EJ. Supera self-expanding stents for endovascular treatment of femoropopliteal disease: a review of the clinical evidence. Vasc Health Risk Manag 2015;11:387–95.

20. Werner M, Paetzold A, Banning-Eichenseer U, et al. Treatment of complex atherosclerotic femoropopliteal artery disease with a self-expanding interwoven nitinol stent: midterm results from the Leipzig SUPERA 500 registry. EuroIntervention 2014;10(7):861–8.

21. Scheinert D, Grummt L, Piorkowski M, et al. A novel self-expanding interwoven nitinol stent for complex femoropopliteal lesions: 24-month results of the SUPERA SFA registry. J Endovasc Ther 2011;18(6):745–52.

22. Chan YC, Cheng SW, Ting AC, et al. Primary stenting of femoropopliteal atherosclerotic lesions using new helical interwoven nitinol stents. J Vasc Surg 2014;59(2):384–91.

23. Yamawaki M, Hirano K, Nakano M, et al. Deployment of self-expandable stents for complex proximal superficial femoral artery lesions involving the femoral bifurcation with or without jailed deep femoral artery. Catheter Cardiovasc Interv 2013;81(6):1031–41.

24. Paris C, White C, Collins T, et al. Catheter-based therapy of common femoral artery atherosclerotic disease. Vasc Med 2011;16(2):109–12.

25. Dattilo P, Tsai T, Rogers K, et al. Acute and medium-terms of endovascular therapy of obstructive disease of the common femoral artery. Catheter Cardiovasc Interv 2013;81(6):1013–22.

Current Endovascular Management of Acute Limb Ischemia

Javier A. Valle, MD, MSc, Stephen W. Waldo, MD*

KEYWORDS

- Peripheral artery disease • Peripheral vascular intervention • Acute limb ischemia • Limb salvage

KEY POINTS

- Acute limb ischemia is a vascular emergency, with a variable presentation that can limit and hinder diagnostic certainty.
- Prompt diagnosis and treatment are critical given the morbidity and mortality associated with the condition.
- Multiple approaches exist to manage acute limb ischemia, with emerging and evolving endovascular approaches showing promise and efficacy.
- There is an ongoing need to determine the optimal long-term management of patients with acute limb ischemia after initial reperfusion.

INTRODUCTION

The incidence of acute limb ischemia (ALI) has decreased over time to 26 cases per 100,000 in the United States.[1] However, ALI remains a vascular emergency, and persistent delays in the recognition and management of this condition continue to place patients at risk for limb loss and subsequent adverse events.[2] Accordingly, this report describes and reviews the current understanding and management of ALI, with a focus on endovascular intervention for limb salvage.

DIAGNOSIS

ALI is defined as the rapid development of decreased limb perfusion, resulting in a new or worsening threat to the viability of a limb.[3] The classic symptoms suggestive of ALI are commonly known as the six "Ps": paresthesias, pain, pallor, pulselessness, poikilothermia, and paralysis. However, the presentation of ALI is markedly variable and can include severe rest pain to decrements in sensation. Physical examination

findings consistent with this diagnosis include absent pulses in the distal limb with cool temperature and pale or mottled skin. There can be a clear demarcation in skin color and temperature below the occluded artery, although the absence of this finding does not exclude the diagnosis.

The subtlety in historical and clinical features and the presence of confounding comorbidities can contribute to the difficulty in diagnostic precision for ALI. More specifically, patients may present with concomitant claudication and diabetic peripheral neuropathy that may mimic several of the symptoms and signs outlined above. However, the acuity of symptom onset should suggest the presence of an acute thrombosis within the peripheral vasculature. The sudden decrement in limb perfusion results in acute symptoms, as there has not been sufficient time for collateral vasculature to mature and circumvent the culprit lesion. Traditionally, the development of decreased limb perfusion occurs within 2 weeks, distinguishing it from the natural progression of critical limb ischemia or diabetic peripheral neuropathy.

Disclosures/Conflicts of Interest: S.W. Waldo receives investigator initiated research support from Merck Pharmaceuticals and Cardiovascular Systems Inc.

Division of Cardiology, VA Eastern Colorado Healthcare System, University of Colorado, 1055 Clermont Street, Denver, CO 80220, USA

* Corresponding author. 1055 Clermont Street, Denver, CO 80220

E-mail address: stephen.waldo@ucdenver.edu

Early diagnosis of this condition is critical to reduce the damage to the affected extremity and improve the rates of limb salvage.[4] Once the diagnosis is suspected, the severity of limb ischemia should be determined using the Rutherford classification (Table 1) to ensure clarity in communication and influence the urgency of revascularization.[5] Classification is determined using physical examination and Doppler pulse evaluation of the affected limb. Patients with class I or IIa limb ischemia may be appropriate for adjunctive diagnostic testing, focused first on delineating anatomy and procedural planning. Duplex ultrasonography, computed tomographic angiography, or magnetic resonance angiography (Fig. 1) can be useful. Echocardiography can also be useful in determining possible embolic sources for ALI but is not as useful in planning revascularization. Ultimately, the gold standard for anatomic evaluation is catheter-based contrast angiography allowing for both diagnostic imaging and direct therapeutic intervention. In patients with class IIb limb ischemia, the limb is acutely threatened, and there is an urgent need for revascularization to maintain tissue viability. In these patients, progression directly to catheter-based angiography is recommended.

ETIOLOGIES

The potential etiologies of ALI are divided into 3 broad categories: (1) thrombosis, (2) trauma/dissection, and (3) embolism. Thrombosis may present suddenly but is also most likely to occur in patients with significant comorbidities (eg, elderly, presence of atherosclerotic cardiovascular disease) at the site of already existing atherosclerotic plaques and may mimic more chronic conditions resulting in delayed presentations. Thrombosis resulting in ALI may also occur in arterial aneurysms, bypass grafts, or endovascular stents. Although thrombotic events in grafts or stents can be related to anatomic or mechanical processes impacting graft or stent function (ie, "kinking" or anastomotic issues in grafts, underexpansion or fracture in stents), they can also occur spontaneously without obvious mechanical issue. In rare cases, hematologic conditions, such as antiphospholipid antibody syndrome or heparin-induced thrombocytopenia, can predispose patients to spontaneous arterial thrombosis in the native vasculature. Trauma can result in severing of the inflow vasculature to the affected limb and is often suggested by history or presentation. Dissection can be spontaneous or trauma-induced and again can be suggested by history and presentation (ie, accidental: gunshot wound, or iatrogenic: recent femoral arterial access). Finally, embolic events can occur from a variety of sources: cardioembolic (left ventricular thrombus, left atrial thrombus in atrial fibrillation, valvular thrombus or pannus), paradoxic emboli, and atheroembolic from more proximal arterial aneurysms with associated thrombus or aortic mural thrombus. Embolic events tend to lodge at bifurcations, such as the common femoral bifurcation or the brachial artery bifurcation in the upper extremity (Fig. 2).

INITIAL MANAGEMENT

After identifying a patient with an acute limb, the initial management focuses on preventing the propagation of thrombus and planning for

Table 1
Rutherford classification of acute limb ischemia

Class	Assessment of Limb Viability	Physical Findings	Pulses
I	Limb viable, no immediate threat	Motor: intact strength Sensory: intact sensation	Arterial: + Doppler Venous: + Doppler
II	Limb threatened		
IIa	Threatened, but salvageable if urgent revascularization	Motor: intact strength Sensory: minimal (end digits) or no deficits	Venous: + Doppler Arterial: +/− Doppler
IIb	Threatened, salvageable if immediate revascularization	Motor: Mild/moderate deficit Sensory: +/++ deficits (beyond end digits), rest pain	Venous: + Doppler Arterial: − Doppler
III	Limb irreversibly damaged: tissue loss, permanent nervous damage	Motor: paralysis Sensory: profound deficits	Venous: − Doppler Arterial: − Doppler

Adapted from Rutherford RB, Baker JD, Ernst C, et al. Recommended standards for reports dealing with lower extremity ischemia: revised version. J Vasc Surg 1997;26:518; with permission.

A   **B**

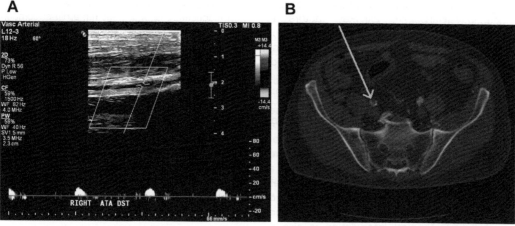

Fig. 1. Diagnostic adjunctive imaging in acute limb ischemia. (A) Duplex ultrasonography and (B) computed tomographic angiographic with an arrow indicating the location of thrombus precipitating acute limb ischemia.

definitive revascularization. Administration of intravenous heparin is recommended to minimize thrombus propagation and should be initiated immediately unless there are active contraindications to anticoagulation (ie, trauma, active bleeding, or suspicion of intracranial hemorrhage). Unfractionated heparin is the agent of choice because of its ability to be monitored and rapid offset if bleeding complications occur, however, should be avoided if heparin-induced thrombocytopenia is suspected. Classification of ALI severity can then guide clinician management with regard to pursuit of further diagnostic

testing versus urgent or emergent revascularization, weighing the risks of limb viability and loss against the benefits of further diagnostic clarity via noninvasive means. In patients with class I ALI (ie, nonthreatened limb), it may be reasonable to pursue a watchful waiting approach with aggressive risk factor modification and initiation of a walking program, with delayed revascularization in the event of symptom persistence. In class II (IIa or IIb) patients, urgent or emergent revascularization is indicated. Finally, in class III patients, in whom limb salvage is impossible, revascularization may actually be harmful, with reperfusion resulting in release of toxic products of metabolism in profound ischemia and muscle infarction like myoglobin, oxygen free radicals, and potassium.[6] In these patients, conservative management or amputation is recommended.[3]

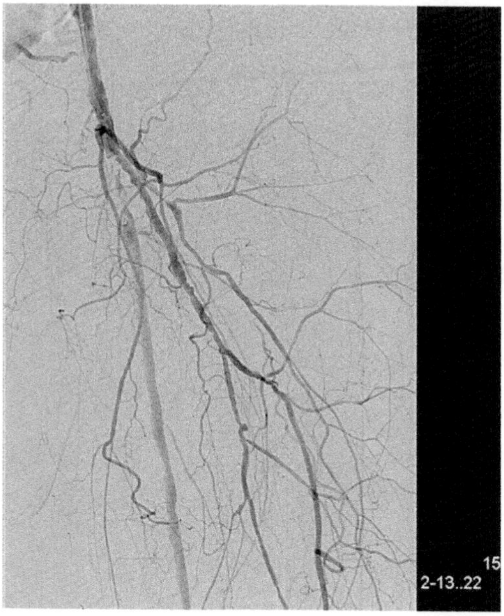

REVASCULARIZATION

Surgical intervention was the traditional method of revascularization for ALI, via surgical (open) thromboembolectomy or arterial bypass. However, catheter-directed thrombolysis, pharmacomechanical thrombolysis, angioplasty, and stenting have offered viable alternatives to open surgical intervention. Patients presenting with this condition have become progressively older, with a higher prevalence of comorbidities, like chronic obstructive pulmonary disease, chronic renal insufficiency, and congestive heart failure, that elevate the perioperative risk of surgical intervention.[1] Clinical trials comparing endovascular and surgical intervention have found similar outcomes between approaches with regard to amputation-free survival and

Fig. 2. Acute limb ischemia resulting from the deposition of thrombus at the bifurcation of the superficial femoral artery and profunda femoris.

overall mortality, despite limitations in the heterogeneity of study populations and endpoints.[7–10] Retrospective studies have found efficacy and safety of endovascular therapies for ALI,[11–13] with some suggesting improved limb salvage and mortality[13] in patients undergoing endovascular therapy, albeit with the caveat of selection bias in observational analyses. These data have driven care toward greater use of endovascular therapy, with an increase in endovascular interventions in the United States from 15.0% to 33.1% from 1998 to 2009,[1] with a recent analysis finding endovascular approaches for ALI to be cost effective when compared with surgical intervention and catheter-directed thrombolysis.[14] Surgical intervention is also a viable treatment option for ALI and should be considered if contraindications to endovascular approaches exist. More specifically, patients with bypass graft infections, contraindication to thrombolytic administration, or patients in whom delays in reperfusion greater than 12 to 24 hours would severely threaten limb viability should be considered for this approach. Surgical and endovascular intervention should thus be viewed as complementary rather than competing approaches for ALI, and hybrid approaches may have a role in certain clinical settings.

ENDOVASCULAR THERAPY

Endovascular therapy for ALI is generally approached in 4 stages: diagnostic angiography, crossing of the lesion, thrombus management (commonly via either elimination or exclusion), and approach to the underlying lesion (angioplasty and stenting). The goal is prompt reperfusion of the affected limb, which generally relies on the use of thrombolytic administration, either in isolation or in conjunction with a mechanical device for aspiration or fragmentation of thrombus to facilitate thrombolysis, as well as angioplasty and stenting. Risks of endovascular approaches include, but are not limited to, bleeding (generally at the access site), vascular injury (both at the access site and the site of intervention), and distal embolization. Randomized controlled trial data supporting endovascular approaches are mainly limited to catheter-directed thrombolysis,[7–9]; however, use of aforementioned adjunctive mechanical therapies has increased over time despite a relative absence of prospective data and is supported by observational analyses.[15]

Diagnostic Angiography
Initial diagnostic imaging should be obtained, ideally with imaging of both inflow and runoff.

Common practice has centered on starting with aorto-iliac imaging for lower extremity ALI to identify any possible distal aortic or aorto-iliac sources for distal embolization, followed by dedicated lower extremity imaging using a support catheter or guiding sheath advanced near the area of interest. Diagnostic angiography should focus not just on identifying the lesion itself, but identifying possible proximal sources of thromboembolism (ie, aortic mural thrombus or aneurysms) and delineating the distal vasculature, including sites of reconstitution, prominent collaterals (if present), and patency below the area of proximal occlusion (**Fig. 3**).

Lesion Crossing
Anticoagulation should be administered to achieve a goal activated clotting time of at least 250 seconds. A guiding catheter should be used to maximize support and allow for device delivery, and use of a support catheter can assist in directionality of wire for lesion crossing. Wire choice depends on the nature of the occlusion. Depending on the chronicity of the lesion, there may be organized or fresh thrombus. An initial strategy of using hydrophilic wires like the Glidewire guidewires (Terumo Interventional) for initial probing of the lesion followed by successive wire escalation to higher tip-loaded wires is recommended. Initial use of hydrophilic wires can allow for "J-ing" or "knuckling" of the wire to allow for increased push while maintaining position within the vessel architecture (**Fig. 4**).

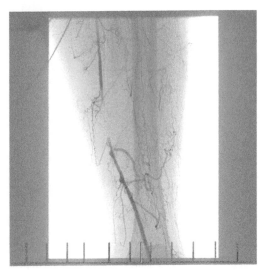

Fig. 3. Diagnostic peripheral angiography shows the presence of collateralization and distal reconstitution.

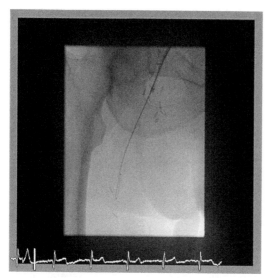

Fig. 4. Recanalization of a thrombotic superficial femoral artery using knuckling of wire.

Thrombus Management—Thrombolysis

Once across the lesion, thrombolytics can be used to modify and debulk the thrombus burden. A sidehole infusion catheter is advanced across the lesion and thrombolytic infused through the catheter. Agents most commonly used are alteplase (Genentech, South San Francisco, CA), reteplase (EKR Therapeutics, Cedar Knolls, NJ), and tenecteplase (Genentech), all variations of recombinant tissue plasminogen activators. Prior agents like urokinase and streptokinase are no longer in favor, with data suggesting more rapid thrombus clearing and less hemorrhage with intra-arterial recombinant tissue plasminogen activator therapy.[16] Duration and volume vary significantly across protocols. Evaluation of high-dose or forced infusion techniques showed achievement of vessel patency in less time but with higher rates of bleeding complications than low-dose infusion and without any significant difference in patency rate or limb salvage at 30 days.[17] However, the patient must be considered in relation to the thrombolytic modality. Prolonged thrombolytic administration (ie, with low-dose infusion) requires prolonged immobility and bed rest, with risk of catheter dislodgement and access site bleeding. Combinations of forced infusion with subsequent low-dose infusion may decrease time required for thrombolytic administration. Additionally, mechanical adjuncts to pharmacologic thrombolysis have been developed, which also may assist in achieving vessel patency more expediently. Distal embolization remains a concern with thrombolytic administration; however, with longer infusion, the thrombolytic is felt to assist in lysing distal emboli as well.

Thrombus Management—Mechanical Adjuncts

Mechanical adjuncts to thrombolysis are divided into 3 major groups: aspiration, rheolytic, and ultrasonic. This review discusses a currently available example of each, understanding that ongoing development will likely lead to further variations and devices offered for use. Benefits of these adjunctive therapies are more rapid recanalization, but may have an attendant increased risk of distal embolization. To maintain the potential benefit of decreasing thrombolytic infusion time, we recommend the use of embolic protection devices, especially in the setting of compromised distal vasculature (ie, single vessel infrapopliteal runoff) to avoid jeopardizing flow distally.

Aspiration thrombectomy is the simplest concept, delivering an open-mouthed catheter over the guidewire to the site of thrombus burden and using a syringe placed at negative pressure to aspirate blood and thrombus particles through the catheter and out of the body. The most common systems require a 6F sheath and use 0.014 wires for delivery. Aspiration thrombectomy is most effective in the absence of large thrombus burden so may not be as useful before significant thrombolysis or in large vessel occlusions. Unfortunately, although aspiration thrombectomy catheters have been studied in the coronary vasculature, their use has not been prospectively validated in the peripheral vasculature. Furthermore, with recent analyses in the coronary literature suggestive of increased embolic events with routine aspiration thrombectomy, there may be similar risks of further embolism in the peripheral vasculature.[18,19]

Rheolytic thrombectomy (Angiojet, Boston Scientific, Marlborough, MA) utilizes a hydrodynamic aspiration mechanism, using high-speed saline jets injected through the catheter tip to create a venturi effect, creating a low-pressure zone and vacuum effect to simultaneously lyse and aspirate thrombus. There are multiple catheter sizes and delivery systems available, ranging from 4F to 6F, using either 0.014 or 0.035 wires also with the capability of delivering thrombolytic through pulse injection. These catheters are over the wire and offer the convenience of combining thrombolysis with mechanical methods of clearing thrombus. Rheolytic thrombectomy has been evaluated in the peripheral vasculature, both with and without pharmacologic thrombolysis, with efficacy ranging from 75% to 90% for recanalization.[20–22]

Therapeutic ultrasound scan can also be used as an adjunct to thrombolytic administration, using high-frequency, low-energy ultrasound waves to accelerate the contact of the pharmacologic thrombolytic with the plasminogen receptor sites within the thrombus. The ultrasound waves both facilitate delivery of the lytic agent and separate the fibrin strands within the thrombus to create a larger surface area on which the agent can act. Ultrasound waves are delivered through an ultrasound core wire, which is inserted through an infusion catheter (EkoSonic Endovascular System, EKOS Corporation, BTG Interventional Medicine, London, UK). When compared with standard catheter-directed thrombolysis, technical success and 30-day patency were similar between methods but with faster thrombolysis and with less thrombolytic administration.[23]

Finally, laser thrombectomy is also a possible mechanical adjunct or stand-alone method of thrombus management, although the supportive data in the peripheral vasculature have been mainly limited to atherectomy and debulking.[24] Excimer laser atherectomy catheters (Turbo-Elite Laser atherectomy catheter, Spectranetics, Inc., Colorado Springs, CO) emit intense bursts of ultraviolet energy in short bursts, or pulses, with a shallow penetration depth to provide focal energy delivery and ablate tissue using a photochemical process, as opposed to hot-tipped lasers that caused high complication rates. Although data supporting laser thrombectomy are limited in the periphery,[25] data exist for its use in the coronary literature.[26]

Thrombus Management—Exclusion

In cases of residual significant thrombus despite aggressive measures to reduce the overall burden, consideration must be given to thrombus exclusion using a covered stent. Polytetrafluoroethylene stent grafts have been used in endovascular treatment of aneurysms with associated thrombus,[27] and a similar strategy can be used in cases of recalcitrant and persistent thrombus in the affected vessel. By excluding the thrombus and presumed underlying thrombogenic lesion from the vessel lumen, one can theoretically arrest further propagation. However, data to support this practice are limited and the recommendation is based mainly on extrapolation.

Approach to the Underlying Lesion

An advantage of thrombus management, in addition to minimizing the possibility of further propagation, is the identification of an underlying lesion that may be responsible or have contributed to the initial thrombosis. Correction either by surgical (ie, graft anastomosis revision) or percutaneous means (balloon angioplasty, drug-coated balloon angioplasty, or stenting) should be pursued. Inability to identify or treat a responsible lesion may predict reocclusion within 6 months.[28] Rationale for interventional approach depends on the findings, with endovascular approaches preferred but not universally applicable.

REPERFUSION

Reperfusion is not a benign process, however, and clinicians should be aware of the potential complications facing patients after restoration of blood flow to an ischemic limb. Ischemia-reperfusion injury can manifest several conditions, including but not limited to swelling of the limb and compartmental pressure elevation. These conditions may be associated with severe pain, paresthesias, and motor dysfunction, with pressure elevations of greater than 30 mm Hg or within 30 mm Hg of diastolic systemic pressure confirming the presence of compartment syndrome that may require surgical fasciotomy. Rates of compartment syndrome after ALI reperfusion can approach up to 20% in some series.[29] Furthermore, release of cytokines and toxic metabolites like myoglobin and potassium from infarcted muscle can result in both hemodynamic instability and renal dysfunction up to and including requirement of hemodialysis.[30] Treatment of these complications is generally supportive, with vascular surgical consultation for measurement of compartmental pressures and aggressive hydration and consultation with nephrology for renal injury.

LONG-TERM MANAGEMENT

Very little data exist to determine the optimal antithrombotic and anticoagulant strategy for patients after an episode of acute limb ischemia. Much depends on both the clinical state of the patient and the etiology of the ischemic event itself. In embolic events, long-term anticoagulation is reasonable, but whether there is differential efficacy between anticoagulation with warfarin or the newer direct oral anticoagulants, like rivaroxaban and apixaban, remains unknown. Antiplatelet therapy with at least aspirin is warranted; however, whether dual antiplatelet therapy should be initiated is similarly unclear, as is duration of therapy. Finally, although there is a suggestion that protease-activated receptor 1 antagonism with vorapaxar may be effective in reducing ALI rates among patients with symptomatic peripheral artery disease,[31] evidence supporting its use after ALI has occurred is nonexistent. Further study is needed to determine an optimal strategy for medical management after episodes of ALI.

SUMMARY

ALI is a vascular emergency, with a variable presentation that can limit and hinder diagnostic certainty. However, prompt diagnosis and treatment is critical given the morbidity and mortality associated with the condition. Multiple approaches exist to manage ALI, with emerging and evolving endovascular approaches showing promise and efficacy. There is an ongoing need, however, to determine the optimal long-term treatment of patients with acute limb ischemia after initial reperfusion.

REFERENCES

1. Baril DT, Ghosh K, Rosen AB. Trends in the incidence, treatment, and outcomes of acute lower extremity ischemia in the United States Medicare population. J Vasc Surg 2014;60:669–77.e2.
2. Brearley S. Acute leg ischaemia. BMJ 2013;346: f2681.
3. Norgren L, Hiatt WR, Dormandy JA, et al. Inter-Society Consensus for the management of peripheral arterial disease (TASC II). Eur J Vasc Endovasc Surg 2007;33(Suppl 1):S1–75.
4. Jivegard L, Holm J, Schersten T. Acute limb ischemia due to arterial embolism or thrombosis: influence of limb ischemia versus pre-existing cardiac disease on postoperative mortality rate. J Cardiovasc Surg 1988;29:32–6.
5. Rutherford RB, Baker JD, Ernst C, et al. Recommended standards for reports dealing with lower extremity ischemia: revised version. J Vasc Surg 1997;26:517–38.
6. Eliason JL, Wakefield TW. Metabolic consequences of acute limb ischemia and their clinical implications. Semin Vasc Surg 2009;22:29–33.
7. Ouriel K, Shortell CK, DeWeese JA, et al. A comparison of thrombolytic therapy with operative revascularization in the initial treatment of acute peripheral arterial ischemia. J Vasc Surg 1994;19:1021–30.
8. Ouriel K, Veith FJ, Sasahara AA. A comparison of recombinant urokinase with vascular surgery as initial treatment for acute arterial occlusion of the legs. Thrombolysis or Peripheral Arterial Surgery (TOPAS) Investigators. N Engl J Med 1998;338:1105–11.
9. Results of a prospective randomized trial evaluating surgery versus thrombolysis for ischemia of the lower extremity. The STILE trial. Ann Surg 1994;220:251–66 [discussion: 266–8].
10. Han SM, Weaver FA, Comerota AJ, et al. Efficacy and safety of alfimeprase in patients with acute peripheral arterial occlusion (PAO). J Vasc Surg 2010; 51:600–9.
11. Earnshaw JJ, Whitman B, Foy C. National Audit of Thrombolysis for Acute Leg Ischemia (NATALI): clinical factors associated with early outcome. J Vasc Surg 2004;39:1018–25.
12. Kashyap VS, Gilani R, Bena JF, et al. Endovascular therapy for acute limb ischemia. J Vasc Surg 2011; 53:340–6.
13. Taha AG, Byrne RM, Avgerinos ED, et al. Comparative effectiveness of endovascular versus surgical revascularization for acute lower extremity ischemia. J Vasc Surg 2015;61:147–54.
14. Vaidya V, Gangan N, Comerota A, et al. Cost-effectiveness analysis of initial treatment strategies for nonembolic acute limb ischemia using real word data. Ann Vasc Surg 2016. [Epub ahead of print].
15. Korabathina R, Weintraub AR, Price LL, et al. Twenty-year analysis of trends in the incidence and in-hospital mortality for lower-extremity arterial thromboembolism. Circulation 2013;128:115–21.
16. Robertson I, Kessel DO, Berridge DC. Fibrinolytic agents for peripheral arterial occlusion. Cochrane Database Syst Rev 2013;(12):CD001099.
17. Kessel DO, Berridge DC, Robertson I. Infusion techniques for peripheral arterial thrombolysis. Cochrane Database Syst Rev 2004;(1):CD000985.
18. Fröbert O, Lagerqvist B, Olivecrona GK, et al. Thrombus aspiration during ST-Segment elevation myocardial infarction. N Engl J Med 2013;369: 1587–97.
19. Jolly SS, Cairns JA, Yusuf S, et al. Randomized trial of primary PCI with or without routine manual thrombectomy. N Engl J Med 2015;372:1389–98.
20. Muller-Hulsbeck S, Kalinowski M, Heller M, et al. Rheolytic hydrodynamic thrombectomy for percutaneous treatment of acutely occluded infra-aortic native arteries and bypass grafts: midterm follow-up results. Invest Radiol 2000;35:131–40.
21. Kasirajan K, Gray B, Beavers FP, et al. Rheolytic thrombectomy in the management of acute and subacute limb-threatening ischemia. J Vasc Interv Radiol 2001;12:413–21.
22. Allie DE, Hebert CJ, Lirtzman MD, et al. Novel simultaneous combination chemical thrombolysis/rheolytic thrombectomy therapy for acute critical limb ischemia: the power-pulse spray technique. Catheter Cardiovasc Interv 2004;63:512–22.
23. Schrijver AM, van Leersum M, Fioole B, et al. Dutch randomized trial comparing standard catheter-directed thrombolysis and ultrasound-accelerated

thrombolysis for arterial thromboembolic infrain-guinal disease (DUET). J Endovasc Ther 2015;22: 87–95.

24. Scheinert D, Laird JR Jr, Schroder M, et al. Excimer laser-assisted recanalization of long, chronic superficial femoral artery occlusions. J Endovasc Ther 2001;8:156–66.

25. Dahm JB, Ruppert J, Doerr M, et al. Percutaneous laser-facilitated thrombectomy: an innovative, easily applied, and effective therapeutic option for recanalization of acute and subacute thrombotic hemodialysis shunt occlusions. J Endovasc Ther 2006;13:603–8.

26. Ambrosini V, Cioppa A, Salemme L, et al. Excimer laser in acute myocardial infarction: single centre experience on 66 patients. Int J Cardiol 2008;127: 98–102.

27. Rajasinghe HA, Tzilinis A, Keller T, et al. Endovascular exclusion of popliteal artery aneurysms with expanded polytetrafluoroethylene stent-grafts: early results. Vasc Endovascular Surg 2006;40:460–6.

28. McNamara TO, Bomberger RA. Factors affecting initial and 6 month patency rates after intraarterial thrombolysis with high dose urokinase. Am J Surg 1986;152:709–12.

29. Henke PK. Contemporary management of acute limb ischemia: factors associated with amputation and in-hospital mortality. Semin Vasc Surg 2009;22:34–40.

30. Ascher E, Haimovici H. Haimovici's vascular surgery. Malden (MA): Blackwell Science; 2004.

31. Bonaca MP, Gutierrez JA, Creager MA, et al. Acute limb ischemia and outcomes with vorapaxar in patients with peripheral artery disease: results from the trial to assess the effects of vorapaxar in preventing heart attack and stroke in Patients With Atherosclerosis-Thrombolysis in Myocardial Infarction 50 (TRA2 degrees P-TIMI 50). Circulation 2016;133:997–1005.

Mechanisms Underlying Drug Delivery to Peripheral Arteries

Jun Li, MD[a,b], Rami Tzafriri, PhD[c],
Sandeep M. Patel, MD[a,b], Sahil A. Parikh, MD, FSCAI[d,*]

KEYWORDS

- Peripheral arterial disease • Drug delivery • Drug-eluting stents • Drug-coated balloons

KEY POINTS

- Despite being a contiguous system, there are drastic architectural, ultrastructural, and biophysiological differences between the coronary and peripheral vascular beds.
- The technologies that have been developed to perfect endovascular revascularization in the coronary artery defies a direct application in the peripheral artery arena.
- An understanding of drug delivery mechanisms and the barriers to absorption is imperative in the development and application of devices in the peripheral arteries.
- Current drug delivery devices available for above-knee targets are broader than for below-knee targets; further studies are necessary to comprehend successful delivery in below-knee arteries.

INTRODUCTION

Peripheral artery disease (PAD) affects an estimated 8.5 million Americans over the age of 40, with a global prevalence of approximately 202 million people.[1] The spectrum of clinical manifestations range from asymptomatic ischemia to exercise-induced claudication to critical limb ischemia (CLI). In patients with PAD, approximately 1% to 3% present with CLI, which still carries with it a high morbidity and mortality rate.[2]

Revascularization remains the cornerstone of therapy for limb salvage in patients with CLI. Moreover, patients with lifestyle-limiting claudication despite guideline-directed medical therapy may undergo revascularization to improve their quality of life and functional status.[1] Endovascular revascularization is a suitable approach in patients with favorable anatomy, as well as for those deemed to be high risk for surgical revascularization, and is frequently considered the first option in patients with both claudication and CLI.

As with all endovascular interventions, the act of dilating the blood vessel with a balloon with or without the additional scaffolding of a stent incites a stereotyped vascular response to injury. The mechanical insult causes a thrombotic

Disclosures: Drs J. Li and S.M. Patel report no disclosures. Dr R. Tzafriri is involved in CBSET studies related to the subject matter that were funded by research grants from Biosensors International Group, Boston Scientific, Cardiovascular Systems Inc, W.L. Gore and Associates, Medtronic, and TriReme Medical Inc. Dr S.A. Parikh serves as a consultant for Abbott Vascular, Boston Scientific, Medtronic, and Spectranetics and receives research support from Boston Scientific, Medtronic, and CR Bard.

[a] Division of Cardiovascular Medicine, Department of Interventional Cardiology, Harrington Heart and Vascular Institute, University Hospitals Cleveland Medical Center, 11000 Euclid Avenue, Cleveland, OH 44106, USA; [b] Department of Medicine, Case Western Reserve University School of Medicine, 2109 Adelbert Road, Cleveland, OH 44106, USA; [c] CBSET Inc, 500 Shire Way, Lexington, MA 02421, USA; [d] Endovascular Services, Division of Cardiology, Department of Medicine, Center for Interventional Vascular Therapy, Columbia University Medical Center/NY Presbyterian Hospital, Columbia University College of Physicians and Surgeons, 161 Fort Washington Avenue, New York, NY 10032, USA
* Corresponding author.
E-mail address: sap2196@cumc.columbia.edu

Intervent Cardiol Clin 6 (2017) 197–216
http://dx.doi.org/10.1016/j.iccl.2016.12.004
2211-7458/17/© 2016 Elsevier Inc. All rights reserved.

response with both fibrin-rich thrombi and platelet aggregation, an inflammatory response that includes monocyte adherence and macrophage infiltration, recruitment and stimulation of vascular smooth muscle cells (SMCs), and circumferential remodeling, which results in intimal hyperplasia and clinical restenosis.[3] Local elution of antiproliferative drugs from stents and balloons is widely used to help curb this cascade of maladaptive responses while limiting the risk of systemic toxicity.

CORONARY VERSUS PERIPHERAL ARTERIES

Although parallels exist between the coronary and peripheral vasculature and the available technology for revascularization, it should be recognized that there are intrinsic differences between the 2 vascular systems in their underlying architecture. The archetype of the vascular wall has been well described, with 3 layers known as tunicae (intima, media, and adventitia). Each layer contains distinct cells and extracellular matrix constituents (Table 1), which serve to not only provide the differential functions for each layer, but also allows for a synergistic and regulatory partnership between the two.[4,5] The extracellular matrix is a dynamic and unique entity, differing based on the type of vessel it resides in, the specific tunica that it generates, and the injury that is incurred (pressure or flow, mechanical, and biochemical). This autoregulatory mechanism is vital in vertebrates with fully closed circulatory systems owing to the need to (i) accept high-pressure ejection in the larger arteries and (ii) accept large volume changes in the remainder of the arterial tree with little change in pressure.[6] Furthermore, on a macroscopic level, arteries in the periphery are subject to significantly taxing mechanical forces (eg, flexion, torsion, compression, elongation, and contraction), compared with coronary arteries. These considerations should be recognized in the development of tools used for endovascular revascularization for the coronaries and lower extremities alike.[7]

Throughout the history of coronary revascularization, many vital lessons have been learned that may be relevant to peripheral revascularization. First, the mechanism of balloon angioplasty is to induce vessel injury to achieve acute lumen gain. However, angioplasty alone has been plagued with abrupt vessel closure, as well as vessel recoil, resulting in both acute and late lumen loss. The advent of bare metal stents (BMS) was intended to circumvent some of the shortcomings of balloon angioplasty. Despite the ability of BMS to reduce

initial adverse events, they remain an imperfect solution for late lumen loss owing to development of in-stent restenosis (ISR; Fig. 1). Drug-eluting stents (DES) were thus introduced as a way to decrease ISR.[8] Despite ongoing advancements aimed at improving DES deliverability, efficacy, and safety to devise the "perfect" stent, stent thrombosis and ISR remain rare but vexing complications.[8,9] Bioresorbable vascular scaffolds (BVS) were developed to curtail the incidence of late ISR and to return vasomotor reactivity to injured vessel, although the first-generation iteration of this technology has been beset by an increased rate of scaffold thrombosis.[10,11]

Comparatively, the narrative on endovascular revascularization of peripheral arteries is still in its infancy. Moreover, the management strategy for 1 peripheral vessel cannot simply be applied to all peripheral vessels (eg, iliacs vs tibial arteries). Experience with drug-coated balloons (DCB) in recent trials suggests that femoral arteries are more forgiving to injury and emboli, providing more flexibility in the development of future technologies for this vascular bed. Moreover, there are some empiric observations that further point to differences in the vascular biology of different vascular beds. For example, recent studies have suggested that the migration of femoral artery vascular SMCs is more attenuated by paclitaxel than coronary vascular SMCs.[12] Nonetheless, the difficulties experienced with coronary revascularization including vessel injury, vessel closure, and ISR remain true in the peripheral vasculature. The effective durability of revascularization is directly related to patency rates, which is affected by vessel location, lesion length, occlusion versus stenosis of the artery at presentation, quality of vessel run-off, and patient comorbidities (diabetes mellitus, chronic kidney disease, and smoking).[1] Currently available treatment modalities for endovascular revascularization of the lower extremities include balloon angioplasty, atherectomy (rotational, excisional, directional, and laser), BMS (self-expanding as well as balloon-expandable stents), DES (self-expanding), and DCBs. Herein we review the concept of drug delivery via DES and DCB in peripheral arteries, being mindful of the role that the ultrastructure of the target vessel wall and its burden of disease significantly alter the vascular response to drug delivery.

PRINCIPLES OF VASCULAR DRUG DELIVERY

The advantage of DES and DCB is to provide localized delivery of a drug while limiting the risk

Table 1
The 3 layers of an arterial wall

Layer	Cells	ECM Components	Structure and Interactions	Physiologic Role
Tunica intima	Endothelial cells	Collagen type IV Fibrillin Laminin Elastin	• Endothelial cells produce elastin and attach to basal lamina, which is supported by the IEL • Collagen and fibrillin anchor endothelial cells to IEL	• Plays major role in embryonic vascular pattern, recruitment of SMCs to vascular wall • Important in atherosclerosis and restenosis
Tunica media	SMCs	Elastin Collagen type III	• Elastin arranged in fenestrated sheets (lamellae) • Between sheets are collagen fibers, thin layers of proteoglycan-rich ECMs, and SMCs • Thin elastic fibers connect lamellae into a 3-dimensional continuous network and connect lamellae with SMCs	• Elastin serves as elastic reservoir and distributes stress evenly and onto collagen fibers • Number of lamellar units is directly related to wall tension; number of units in a particular vessel does not change after birth • Mature aorta eliminates SMCs, suggestive that mechanical characteristics are a function of the ECM
Tunica adventitia	Myofibroblasts Progenitor cells[a]	Collagen (types I and III primarily)	• Defined as area outside of EEL • Myofibroblasts produce collagen • Vaso vasorum present in larger mammals with >29 lamellae in tunica media	• Prevents vascular rupture at high pressures • Vasa vasorum provides nourishment and oxygen to cells in the tunica media (owing to inadequate nutrients by translational filtration)

The symbiotic relationship of cells and ECMs within each layer allows for autoregulation and helps drive the physiologic role of each tunica.[4–6]

Abbreviations: ECM, extracellular matrix; EEL, external elastic lamina; IEL, internal elastic lamina; SMCs, smooth muscle cells.

[a] Progenitor cells are capable of differentiating into SMCs.

of systemic toxicities. Given the narrow therapeutic window of some antiproliferative drugs, the extent of drug elution, release kinetics, drug partitioning, specific and nonspecific tissue binding, and net tissue concentration are important properties to consider to prevent localized toxicity but maintain therapeutic efficacy (**Fig. 2**).[13]

Mechanistic computational modeling offers a unified framework by which to evaluate the interplay of these variables with each other and with lesion properties. In reviewing the underlying mechanisms and models, we shall follow the practice of tracking the directed nature of endovascular drug delivery, focusing first on the processes

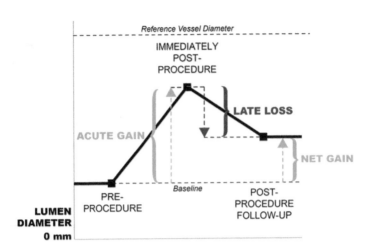

Fig. 1. After angioplasty or placement of a stent, there is an acute gain in lumen size but with vessel recoil and in-stent restenosis (ISR), there is late loss in the vessel diameter, resulting in a net gain that is less than the initially achieved lumen size.

underlying drug release from the surface of the device and then on the processes governing drug absorption and distribution in the arterial wall.[7,14,15]

Drug Classes

The idea of using antiproliferative, immunosuppressants to limit neointimal hyperplasia was adapted from tumor chemotherapy.[16] Importantly, drugs chosen for DES and DCB are typically lipophilic, so as to improve binding to

tissue and passage through cellular membranes.[17] Hydrophilic molecules (eg, heparin) tend to have a higher propensity for blood distribution rather than tissue. Once absorbed into tissue, hydrophilic molecules have a tendency to dwell in the extracellular space rather than move intracellularly, further limiting their ability to exert pharmacologic effects.[17]

The Limus family of drugs includes sirolimus, everolimus, zotarolimus, and biolimus A9.[18] These bind to the intracellular FKBP12 protein receptor

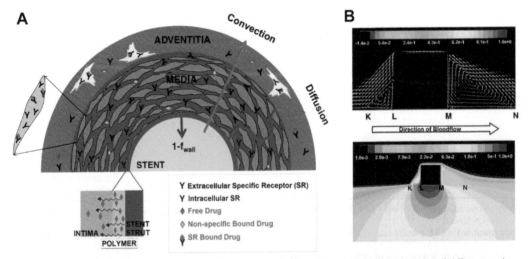

Fig. 2. (A) The processes that determine drug distribution and effect. Governed by the principles of diffusion and convection, drugs are transmitted from the polymer overlying the stent strut into the arterial wall owing to concentration and pressure gradients, respectively. Within the arterial wall, there are free drugs and bound drugs (specific receptor binding as well as nonspecific binding to elements of the extracellular matrix). (B) Simulation of fluid dynamics to show the effects that a protruding stent strut has on fluid recirculation (top), which result in asymmetric drug deposition proximal and distal to the stent strut (bottom). This is more important in older generation drug-eluting stents and in current generation bioresorbable vascular scaffolds owing to the thickness of the struts. (Adapted from Tzafriri AR, Groothuis A, et al. Stent elution rate determines drug deposition and receptormediated effects. J Control Release 2012;161:918–26; with permission; and Kolachalama VB, Tzafriri AR, Arifin DY, et al. Luminal flow patterns dictate arterial drug deposition in stent-based delivery. J Control Release 2009;133(1):24–30; with permission.)

in SMCs, which then binds to the signal transduction protein mammalian target of rapamycin, halting cell cycle progression at the G1/S phase and resulting in cytostatic effects (Fig. 3).[16,18] Sirolimus, also known as rapamycin, is a macrolide compound produced by the bacterium *Streptomyces hygroscopicus*. Cypher (Cordis Corporation, Milpitas, CA), with the use of sirolimus, was the first polymer-coated coronary DES to gain both the Conformité Européenne mark and US Food and Drug Administration (FDA) approval.[18]

The non-Limus alternative is paclitaxel of the taxane class. Its mechanism of action is through the interruption of microtubule assembly in the S/G2/M phase of the cell cycle, resulting in cytotoxic effects (see Fig. 3).[16] Cytotoxicity may result in the theoretic disadvantage of inducing necrosis and increasing inflammation, although it has been speculated that paclitaxel may be primarily cytostatic at lower concentrations.[16] Taxus, a paclitaxel-eluting stent, was the second DES to receive FDA approval for coronary revascularization. Current FDA approved DES and DCB for peripheral arteries use paclitaxel as the antiproliferative drug.

Drug Delivery Mechanisms

Diffusion is the dominant mechanism for controlled drug release from stents, although other proposed mechanisms include dissolution, erosion, ion exchange, and antibody binding (Table 2).[17] In diffusion-controlled release, drugs are maintained on the delivery device by either a reservoir system or monolithic system (Fig. 4). In the reservoir system, drug is loaded as a distinct phase and its rate of release is controlled by the rate of solubilization (eg, hydrophobic drugs) or

via an external membrane that serves as the main diffusion barrier.[19] Theoretically, the use of a rate-limiting membrane in reservoir designs can result in a constant release rate, or zero-order kinetics, by which the rate of release is determined by device surface area in contact with the biological surface.[17,19] There is a risk of "dose dumping" owing to membrane rupture in this system.[19] Nonpolymer coated DES such as the Zilver PTX (Cook Medical, Bloomington, IN) and Biofreedom stents (Biosensors International, Singapore) do not use a rate-limiting membrane, yet are able to sustain therapeutic tissue levels via slow solubilization and/or protein binding interactions.

In the monolithic or matrix system, drugs are imbedded within a polymer coating that serves as the diffusion barrier.[17,19] The matrix may be nonporous/homogeneous, in which there is only 1 phase through which the drug diffuses, or porous/granular, whereby diffusion can only occur at the pores and the matrix is otherwise impermeable.[19]

Whereas stents can provide a scaffold for sustained intravascular drug elution, DCBs are only inflated for a matter of minutes and typically deliver their drug load as part of a coating that is transferred or "painted" onto the blood–tissue interface (Fig. 5). Different coatings transfer by a range of mechanisms, either as embolized or preformed drug-laden particulates or as islands that "paint" contiguous areas on the tissue surface. As a result, compared with DES, delivery by DCB is more variable and relies on additional forces to retain the delivered drug at the target tissue. Alternative, drug-eluting balloons and catheters use a convective pressure

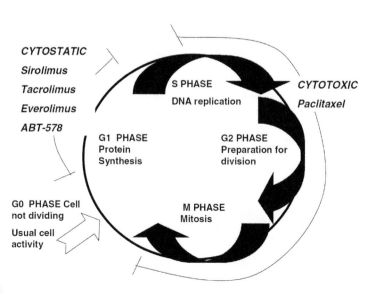

CYTOSTATIC
Sirolimus
Tacrolimus
Everolimus
ABT-578

S PHASE
DNA replication

CYTOTOXIC
Paclitaxel

G1 PHASE
Protein
Synthesis

G2 PHASE
Preparation for
division

G0 PHASE Cell
not dividing

Usual cell
activity

M PHASE
Mitosis

Fig. 3. The cell cycle with the mode of action of antiproliferative drugs used in drug-eluting stents and drug-coated balloons. (*From* Smith EJ, Rothman MT. Antiproliferative coatings for the treatment of coronary heart disease. J Interv Cardiol 2003;16:476; with permission.)

Table 2
Proposed mechanisms for controlling endovascular drug release

Mechanism	Conditions	Design Parameters
Diffusion	Drug must be mobile within coating or reservoir	• Drug size • Lipophilicity • Loading gradients • Polymer composition • Molecular weight
Dissolution	Solid drug particles must dissolve before drug diffusion	• Drug particle size and solubility • Reservoir volume • Water accessibility
Erosion	Polymer erosion increases the mobility of trapped drug	• Polymer type • Molecular weight • Glass transition temperature • Drug size • Drug lipophilicity
Ion exchange	Charged drug, oppositely charged device-surface groups	• Ratio of drug load to surface charge density
Antibody binding	Drug binds to device-surface epitopes	• Ratio of drug load to surface binding sites

Adapted from Tzafriri AR, Edelman ER. Endovascular drug delivery and drug elution systems. Interv Cardiol Clin 2016;5:307–20; with permission.

to transfer drug solutions, dispersions, or drug-loaded nanoparticles.

Although the concept of the DCB has been long established, perfecting DCB performance proved challenging. Of critical importance was the identification of appropriate drugs that could be transiently bound to the balloon and then released into the vascular wall, as well as the development of techniques for preventing extraneous loss to the bloodstream during transport to and from the target lesion and to deliver an adequate amount of drug at the target lesion during short inflations. An important breakthrough was the realization that excipients can both help to bind the drug to the balloon surface and assists with transfer onto the arterial wall (Box 1).

The initial emergence of paclitaxel as a plausible candidate for balloon-based drug delivery was based on its lipophilicity and its sustained inhibition (for days) of vascular SMC proliferation after short exposure times (seconds to minutes).[20–22] This concept was first illustrated in porcine arteries injected with contrast medium containing paclitaxel and also in porcine arteries that underwent paclitaxel-coated balloon (PCB) angioplasty.[21,23–25]

In a proof-of-concept study, Scheller and colleagues[23] used BMS mounted atop PCB to evaluate the loss of paclitaxel in blood with routine transport and retention of drug in coronary arteries of domestic pigs. BMS mounted on standard balloons served as the control arm. Two different excipients and coating processes were used in this study (ethyl acetate with a drug concentration of 2 µg/mm^2 and acetone with a drug concentration of either 1.3 or 2.5 µg/mm^2). The authors estimated that PCBs lose approximately 6% of its dose with delivery to the coronary arteries and back, and approximately 80% of the drug is released with inflation.[23] Neointimal proliferation was reduced significantly in PCBs coated using acetone but not in those with ethyl acetate. This difference was attributed to the presence of hydrophilic x-ray contrast-medium substance in the coating

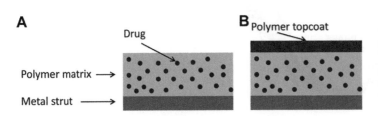

Fig. 4. Schematics of a monolithic (A) and reservoir (B) drug-coating systems on stents. (Adapted from Tzafriri AR, Edelman ER. Endovascular drug delivery and drug elution systems. Interv Cardiol Clin 2016;5:312; with permission.)

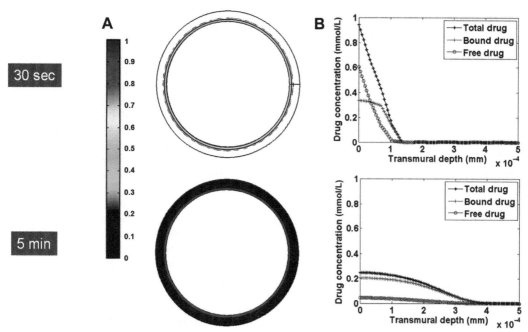

Fig. 5. Computational mapping of zotarolimus arterial distribution after delivery with drug-coated balloon inflation for 30 seconds. (*A*) Schematic showing the total drug concentration at 30 seconds and 5 minutes after inflation. (*B*) At 30 seconds, the total, bound, and free drugs are maximal at the mural surface; at 5 minutes, there is distribution across the arterial wall, with a peak drug concentration of approximately 25% of the peak at 30 seconds. Note that the drug is predominantly bound at 5 minutes. (*Adapted from* Kolachalama VB, Pacetti SD, Franses JW, et al. Mechanisms of tissue uptake and retention in zotarolimus-coated balloon therapy. Circulation 2013;127:2047–55; and Tzafriri, Edelman. Biomaterials Forum. 2016 (Third Quarter). p. 13.)

preparation of the former, suggesting that the biochemical properties of excipients play a vital role in the efficacy of drug transport in DCBs.[23,26] At present, the preferred excipients for DCBs are nonpolymeric carriers (usually hydrophilic) that help to provide a uniform coating and enhance the transfer of lipophilic drugs onto the arterial wall.[27]

Endovascular Diffusion Barriers to Drug Absorption

Although the endothelium can limit drug absorption,[14,15] it is typically disrupted in atherosclerotic lesions; when present, it is denuded during angioplasty. The presence of atherosclerosis, calcium, thrombus, and intimal hyperplasia can impede the distribution of drug into the arterial wall.[28] Tzafriri and colleagues[28] performed an ex vivo study of paclitaxel distribution using both human autopsy abdominal aorta as well as rabbit arteries subjected to diet control and catheter-induced vascular injury. The authors used a controlled mechanism of drug delivery via prolonged incubation in static drug-binding media, with the notion that the immersion of arteries in drug-binding media circumvents any irregularity in

drug delivery owing to stent deployment technique and stent geometry. In control arteries from animals fed on a normal diet, it was demonstrated that paclitaxel uptake largely tracked elastin lamella, similar to reports on model hydrophilic drugs.[7,29,30] Owing to the small size of paclitaxel relative to elastin fenestrations, this barrier effect of elastin has been attributed to hydrophobic binding and directly illustrated in artificial tissue mimics.[31] The hydrophobic nature of paclitaxel also dictates a greater affinity for lipids in tissue, prompting some to suggest that partitioning of paclitaxel and sirolimus analogues should scale positively with lipid content. Although such a trend has been demonstrated for model hydrophobic drugs in artificial acellular plaques, increased lipid content in arterial tissue displaces other drug-binding elements such as elastin and high-affinity intracellular receptors. Thus, Tzafriri and colleagues[28] reported that paclitaxel distribution is related inversely to lipid content, with increased deposition in regions with tubulin and elastin, but decreased deposition in lipid-rich regions.[28] Interestingly, the authors noted that a diet rich in cholesterol blunted the peak quantity of paclitaxel binding, yet this diet-related difference was not observed in everolimus binding curves. This differential sensitivity to lipid content was attributed to the higher density of paclitaxel receptors (eg, microtubules) relative to sirolimus receptors (eg, FKBP12).

The presence of thrombus after stent implantation has also been implicated in affecting the rate of drug absorption. However, the exact effect of thrombus depends on the diffusivity of drug in the arterial wall versus in thrombus, as determined by the unique physicochemical properties of each drug within each realm.[32] For a drug with higher diffusivity in the arterial wall compared with thrombus, it is sequestered in the thrombus. This increases the availability of drug for transport into the arterial wall in a slow-release fashion and ultimately increases drug deposition. Conversely, if the diffusivity of a drug is higher in thrombus compared with the arterial wall, there will be no thrombus-related alteration in drug absorption.[32]

Last, in the case of ISR, the pathologic substrate is primary composed of hypocellular and fibrotic inflammatory tissue rich in proteoglycans. Typically this is the result of SMC proliferation, although in some patients, evidence of neoatherosclerosis can be appreciated on intravascular imaging.[33] Without appropriate ablation and modification of this tissue before the deployment of either a DES or DCB, drug delivery to the underlying arterial wall may be hindered. The issue of ablative therapy for ISR is discussed in detail elsewhere in this article.

Drug Dynamics in the Arterial Wall

Once within the wall, drugs exist in either a solid form, a soluble form, or a bound form (see Fig. 2). Because the drug is inert in its solid form, dissolution is an important process of lipophilic drugs, particularly for DCB and DES that deliver their load in particulate forms. Solubilized drug molecules distribute in the tissue by a combination of convective transport along the radial pressure gradient and diffusive transport along concentration gradients. Tissue ultrastructure and density impact both these processes as molecular transport occurs through macropores and micropores in the tissue. Importantly, convection and diffusion are both retarded with increasing molecular weight, but in a manner that favors convection. Thus, arterial wall distribution of coating particles and drug-laden nanoparticles occurs primarily via convection and is therefore sensitive to arterial pressure and benefits from intravascular delivery.[14,34,35]

Solubilized drug can also bind to extracellular proteins and lipids, as well as to intracellular molecules. By sequestering the drug, the binders effectively slow the distribution of the drug but also increase the capacity of the tissue to absorb and retain drug. Although mutual affinity dictates the strength of interaction between a single drug molecule and a single binding site, a tissue's binding potential for a drug scales as the product of the affinity and the density of binding sites. Thus, although a drug's affinity for a receptor is high relative to its affinity to hydrophobic binding sites within the tissue, the degree by which either of these binding processes impedes drug distribution and sustains tissue distribution is also determined by the relative expression of these binding sites, which can vary with artery type. Experimental evidence suggests that the density of nonspecific binding sites greatly exceeds the density of sirolimus receptors in arterial tissue,[36] but is comparable with the density of paclitaxel receptors.[36,37] This difference is particularly important for DCBs and fast eluting stents that rely on binding to retain the delivered drug within the lesion.[38,39] Although it has been argued that the expression of sirolimus receptors in the arterial wall of coronary arteries is sufficiently high to retain sirolimus analogues long after release from stents (Fig. 6), it is intriguing to speculate that the greater efficacy of paclitaxel-eluting stents versus sirolimus-eluting stents (SES) in peripheral arteries (but not in coronary arteries) might be explained partially by higher paclitaxel binding potential of peripheral versus coronary arteries.

Whereas the basic concepts of balloon-based drug delivery are known, mechanistic quantitative studies of these processes are rare compared with the rich literature on drug-eluting stents. An exception to this is the in vitro, in silico, and in vivo study performed by Kolachalama and colleagues[39] on zotarolimus-eluting balloons and PCBs, which effectively illustrates several key concepts on this technology. First, only an estimated 2% of total drug, and 24% of releasable drug is transferred within the first 30 seconds of inflation. The release follows a first-order kinetics, reaching steady state at approximately 5 minutes after inflation.[39] The balloon inflation provides bulk transfer of the drug onto the mural surface, with a subsequent transport within the arterial wall via diffusion and reversible binding.[40] As expected, a longer inflation time (ie, 180 seconds vs 30 seconds) resulted in increased tissue uptake both with computational modeling and in vivo

data.[39] Finally, using computational modeling and intravascular ultrasound–virtual histology to determine vessel-specific constituents, Mandal and colleagues[41] showed that heterogeneity in tissue composition dictates drug retention rates. This finding is consistent with previous observations that diffusion barriers can affect the true deposition and transport of drug when tissue is heterogeneous, as is the case in a "real-world" application of DCB. Given that the presence of lipid deposits and calcific lesions will hinder drug absorption, ample lesion preparation and possibly debulking is essential to assist in drug delivery.[42,43] The role of atherectomy in clinical practice is described in detail elsewhere in this article.

Experience with PCBs has shown that the morphology of coating is vital to drug delivery efficacy and performance.[27,44] First-generation PCBs had a high level of crystallinity on the coating surface, which resulted in inconsistent drug load and increased particulate shedding during balloon inflation (Fig. 7).[45,46] The amorphous coating allows for more uniform distribution of the drug. However, based on an animal study from Granada and colleagues,[45] this type of coating was found to have drastically lower drug retention within the arterial wall at greater than 24 hours compared with crystalline coating, despite achieving similar initial deposition levels at 1 hour after inflation. Furthermore, postmortem histologic assessments of porcine coronary arteries showed increased neointimal

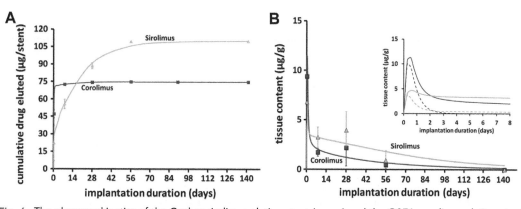

Fig. 6. The pharmacokinetics of the Cypher sirolimus-eluting stent (*green*) and the O3FA corolimus-eluting stent (*red*), which is a uniquely developed drug-eluting stent with cross-linked omega-3 fatty acid based coating that is 85% absorbed and elutes 97% of its drug within 8 days of implantation. Despite fast elution by the O3FA coating, there is sustained tissue retention owing to the presence of nonspecific receptor binding. (*A*) In vivo release kinetics for both stents. (*B*) In vivo tissue content (*symbols*) is closely predicted by computational model (*lines*) that account for the high affinity drug binding to FKBP12. Inset illustrates the early tissue content in the first few days after implantation; here, simulation (*solid lines*) do not account for high affinity drug binding to FKBP12 (*dashes*). (*Adapted from* Artzi N, Tzafriri AR, Faucher KM, et al. Sustained efficacy and arterial drug retention by a fast drug eluting cross-linked fatty acid coronary stent coating. Ann Biomed Eng 2016;44:282; with permission.)

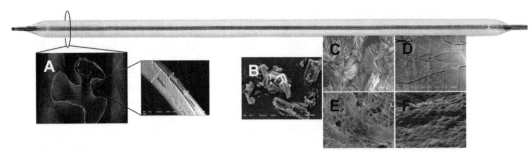

Fig. 7. The anatomy of a drug-coated balloon (DCB) as visualized by surface electron microscopy. (*A*) A DCB cut in cross-section, with the inlet showing close of the balloon and its adherent coating. (*B*) Anhydrous crystal of paclitaxel. Types of coating as the result of different excipients and processing methods, shown as (*C*) crystalline, (*D*) amorphous, (*E*) hybrid, and (*F*) nanospheres. (*Adapted from* Granada JF. Technical and biologic challenges for future DCB development. 2nd International DEB Symposium. 2012.)

hyperplasia with amorphous coating compared with crystalline coating.[45] Other forms of coating morphologies have been developed to try to maximize drug delivery but at the same time limit inconsistent retention and distribution (eg, hybrid and nanospheres in Fig. 7).[46,47]

CLINICAL APPLICATIONS
Stent-Based Delivery
The 3 primary constituents of DES that govern the deliverability, efficacy, and safety of the device are stent platform, polymer coating, and drug. The interplay among these 3 components is unique for each stent, and requires extensive in vitro as well as in vivo testing to clearly determine the integrated effect on vessel response to injury.[36] The underlying platform may be metallic or polymeric (in the case of BVS) and serve as a framework for artery structure after injury is induced by angioplasty, as well as a drug delivery vehicle to localize the distribution of drugs. We review the available clinical trials on several DES that have been developed for use in peripheral arteries. Currently, Zilver PTX is the only FDA-approved DES available for implantation in the femoropopliteal artery.

Stent-Based Delivery in the Superficial Femoral Artery: The Limus Family
The first study investigating the use of DES in the lower extremities was the SIROCCO trial (Sirolimus Coated Cordis Self-Expandable Stent), which randomized patients to either sirolimus-eluting or bare metal SMART self-expanding nitinol stent (n = 93).[48–50] Enrollment criteria included Rutherford stage 1 to 4 symptoms with de novo or restenotic lesions in the native superficial femoral artery (SFA) with 70% or greater stenosis. Lesion lengths were up to 20 cm in the first phase of the study (SIROCCO I),[48] and 14.5 cm in the second phase (SIROCCO II).[49] In combined data at 24 months, the rate of ISR was similar in both treatment arms (22.9% vs 21.1% in DES vs BMS; P>.05).[50] Nonetheless, target lesion revascularization (TLR) was lower in the sirolimus-eluting group (6% vs 13%, sirolimus-eluting vs bare metal stent), although this difference was also not statistically significant. The authors concluded that DES were a safe and feasible option for treatment of patients with complex and critical lower extremity PAD.[50] As the initial experience with peripheral arterial DES, a great deal of scrutiny was applied to the neutral result. The lack of difference in ISR between the DES and BMS were explained by uncommonly low BMS restenosis rates and suboptimal drug elution in the DES arm, with a low drug load (90 µg/cm^2, akin to coronary dosing) that is largely released within 7 days.[48,50]

The STRIDES (Superficial Femoral Artery Treatment with Drug-Eluting Stents) trial was a nonrandomized, single arm study to evaluate the performance of the Dynalink (Abbott Vascular, Santa Clara, CA) self-expanding nitinol stent with everolimus embedded with ethylene vinyl alcohol copolymer (Dynalink-E stent).[51] Notably, the Dynalink-E stent incorporates a 2.5-fold greater drug load relative to the SMART SES (225 µg/cm^2 vs 90 µg/cm^2).[52] In addition to the increased drug concentration, the elution profile for the Dynalink-E reflects approximately 80% drug release over 90 days (comparatively, in coronary sirolimus-eluting and everolimus-eluting stents (EES) with concentrations of 140 µg/cm^2 and 100 µg/cm^2, respectively, drug release occurs over 30 days).[52] Patients included in the study had Rutherford stage 2 to 5 symptoms with SFA or popliteal lesions 3 to 17 cm in length (n = 104). Primary patency rates, defined as freedom from 50% or greater ISR by duplex evaluation, was 68% at 12 months.[51] This was nominally improved compared with a similar patient population receiving the Dynalink BMS (63%) at 12 months,[52,53] although a head-to-head comparison is needed to confirm this observation.

Taken together, these data suggest that the DES used in SIROCCO and STRIDES were either not implanted with enough drug or that the elution kinetics were not tailored adequately to overcome chronic interactions between the stent and the artery (eg, the chronic outward force exerted on the vessel by a typical self-expanding nitinol stent). At present, in the only large, controlled studies of Limus-eluting DES in the SFA, it seems that there is no significant therapeutic efficacy of the evaluated DES compared with control BMS.

Stent-Based Delivery in the Superficial Femoral Artery: The Taxanes

The largest trial of DES in the peripheral arteries is the Zilver PTX Randomized Clinical Trial that compared a self-expanding, open cell, nitinol DES with polymer-free paclitaxel coating with standard percutaneous transluminal angioplasty (PTA; n = 474).[54] Patient inclusion criteria were Rutherford stage 2 or greater, angiographic stenosis 50% or greater, and lesion length less than or equal to 14 cm, with 1 or more patent runoffs containing less than 50% stenosis throughout. Of the patients randomized to PTA, approximately 50% had acute PTA failure defined as 30% or greater stenosis, 5 mm Hg or greater mean transstenotic pressure gradient, or persistent flow-limiting dissection. Patients with PTA failure required a secondary randomization for provisional DES vs BMS, although the primary analysis at 1 year was performed as an intention-to-treat protocol.[54] Primary patency was determined by a duplex peak systolic velocity ratio of less than 2.0 or angiographic stenosis of less than 50% if available. At 1 year, primary patency (93.1% vs 32.8%, DES vs PTA; P<.001) and clinically driven TLR (9.5% vs 17.5%, DES vs PTA; P = .01) were both significantly better in the DES group.[54] Provisional DES also showed superior primary patency (89.9% vs 73.0%, DES vs BMS; P = .01).[54] These findings were consis-tent at the 2- and 5-year follow-up evaluation.[55,56] At 5 years, the primary patency rates of overall DES (combined primary DES and provisional DES) versus standard care (optimal PTA with or without provisional BMS) was 66.4% versus 43.3% (P<.01).[56] Patients who underwent provisional DES also had improved primary patency rates compared with provisional BMS (72.4% vs 53.0%; P = .03) at 5 years.[56]

The MAJESTIC (Stenting of the Superficial Femoral and/or Proximal Popliteal Artery Project) trial is a recent single-arm study evaluating the use of a drug-eluting self-expanding nitinol stent (Eluvia, Boston Scientific, Marlborough, MA) in patients with Rutherford stage 2 to 4 symptoms and stenosis of 70% or greater or occlusion in a length of 3 to 11 cm (n = 57).[57] The stent platform is based on the Innova stent (Boston Scientific, Marlborough, MA), which contains closed cell end rows for deployment stability and open cell within the stent to maximize flexibility, conformability, and fracture resistance. The drug coating uses a dual layer system, with the primer layer adjacent to the stent, and the active layer on top of the primer. The primer layer promotes adhesion of the active layer to the stent, whereas the active layer contains paclitaxel at a concentration of 0.167 $\mu g/cm^2$.[57,58] At 12 months, primary patency (defined as duplex peak systolic velocity ratio of $\leq$2.5 in the absence of TLR) was 96%, whereas the TLR was 4%.[57]

Although we should be cautious to make a direct comparison between the Zilver PTX and MAJESTIC outcomes owing to differences trial designs, there is a remarkable improvement in primary patency and TLR rates with Eluvia compared with Zilver PTX. There are stark differences in the stent platform design as well as the drug-coating mechanism between the 2 stents; thus, it may be difficult to determine the primary contributor to the noted differences. However, it has been speculated that perhaps a slowly eluting DES may have better outcomes compared with a fast-eluting DES, which in turn performs better than the standard nitinol self-expanding BMS.[59] Indeed, an in vivo pharmacokinetics study of the Zilver PTX stent showed that only 34.3 $\pm$ 4.8% of the initial paclitaxel dose was present on the stent at 0.5 hours after implantation, and 5.2 $\pm$ 4.6% remain at 24 hours.[60] Despite the fast drug delivery from the stent, the drug was sustained in the tissue long after drug elution, declining to minimally detectable levels only after 56 days.[60] Conversely, in the Eluvia stent 27% of the total loading dose was released by day 4, and 73% by day 180.[12] The mean drug concentration at the target tissue ranged from 3.72 ng/mg at 10 days to 0.38 ng/mg at 180 days.[12] The findings of these 2 pharmacokinetics studies have been summarized in **Fig. 8**. The IMPERIAL trial (ELUVIA Drug-eluting Stent vs Zilver PTX Stent) to compare the performance of these

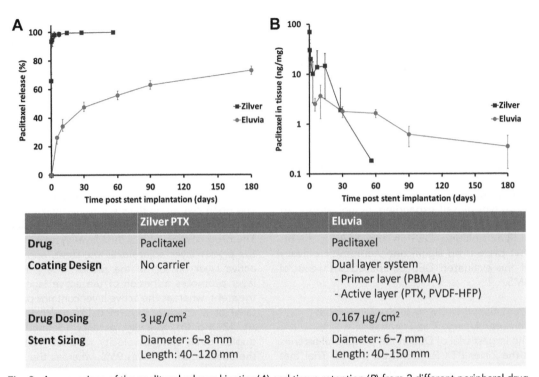

	Zilver PTX	Eluvia
Drug	Paclitaxel	Paclitaxel
Coating Design	No carrier	Dual layer system - Primer layer (PBMA) - Active layer (PTX, PVDF-HFP)
Drug Dosing	3 µg/cm²	0.167 µg/cm²
Stent Sizing	Diameter: 6–8 mm Length: 40–120 mm	Diameter: 6–7 mm Length: 40–150 mm

Fig. 8. A comparison of the paclitaxel release kinetics (A) and tissue retention (B) from 2 different peripheral drug-eluting stents, Zilver PTX and Eluvia, as extrapolated from pharmacokinetics data of each stent.[12,60] The variation in the speed of drug delivery is attributed to the difference in the presence (Eluvia) and absence (Zilver PTX) of a polymer. The presence of a polymer allows paclitaxel to be slowly eluted and absorbed over days to months, extending the duration of effects. (C) The characteristics of Zilver PTX versus Eluvia stents, with highlighted differences in drug dosing and coating designs. The primer layer attaches the active layer to the stent strut.[58] PBMA, poly-n-butyl methacrylate; PTX, paclitaxel; PVDF-HFP, polyvinylidene fluoride co-hexafluoropropylene.

2 stents directly in patients with significant SFA and/or proximal popliteal arteries is currently underway.[58]

Bioresorbable Vascular Scaffolds

The notion of using a BVS in peripheral arteries is an attractive alternative for several reasons. First, any DES ultimately becomes a BMS after drug elution has been completed, rendering the residual device to be a nidus for ongoing chronic inflammation and vascular injury, ultimately resulting in ISR and increased late lumen loss. This is potentiated by stent fracture, which is felt to be more common with metallic scaffolds as opposed to BVS. In addition, BVS has been touted to allow the return of vasomotor function after dissolution of the scaffold, although definite in vivo data of this theoretic advantage are lacking. Furthermore, BVS will allow for adjunctive imaging via computed tomography and MRI of the lower extremity arteries without inflicting metallic artifacts. Last but not least, the implantation of nonmetallic scaffolds obviates the difficulty of surgical anastomosis at the

target vessel in the future should bypass be deemed necessary.

Limited data are currently available on this application. With the use of an absorbable metal stent in patients with CLI (n = 20), Peeters and colleagues[61] demonstrated a primary patency rate of 89.5% at 3 months. More recently, Varcoe and colleagues[62] demonstrated the feasibility of implanting ABSORB everolimus-eluting BVS (Abbott Vascular, Santa Clara, CA) in patients with CLI or severe claudication (n = 14). One patient in the study did suffer acute scaffold thrombosis on postprocedural day 1, which was salvaged with repeat revascularization and implantation of one metallic stent. No further TLR episodes were recorded in this pilot study (median follow-up, 6 months).[62] The ESPRIT I was a first-in-human study that evaluated the use of a BVS (everolimus-eluting poly-L-lactide scaffold) in the external iliac artery and SFA.[63] At 2 years, binary restenosis rate was 16.1% and TLR 11.8%, without any device-related deaths or amputations.[63] An ongoing clinical trial, ABSORB BTK (The ABSORB

Bioresorbable Scaffold Below the Knee Study) from the University of New South Wales is currently recruiting patients.

Drug-Coated Balloons in the Superficial Femoral Artery

Despite promising results for the use of DES in lower extremity revascularization, there remains a prominent risk of biological and mechanical device failure given dynamic mechanical stressors, resulting in long-term restenosis and stent fracture. To date, BVS in the lower extremity has limited experimental applications primarily outside the United States. However, DCBs offer the capability to deliver drug and improve patency rates compared with plain angioplasty but without the liability of long-term commitment to metallic scaffold implantation.

The THUNDER (Local Taxane with Short Exposure for Reduction of Restenosis in Distal Arteries) trial was the first randomized controlled trial to evaluate the use of DCB in the superficial femoral or popliteal artery (n = 154).[20] Patients with symptomatic PAD with Rutherford stage 1 to 5 and greater than 70% stenosis with a length of greater than 2 cm in the SFA or popliteal artery were randomized to one of 3 groups: PCB (concentration 3 µg/mm² embedded in iopromide) and standard contrast medium, standard balloons and paclitaxel in contrast medium, or standard balloons and standard contrast medium.[20] Additional PTA was performed with nonstudy balloon if residual stenosis of greater than 30% was noted; nitinol stent was used as rescue or if ongoing residual stenosis noted. Reduced TLR was noted in the PCB arm versus standard balloon with standard contrast medium at 6 months (4% vs 37%; P<.001) and on 5-year follow-up (21% vs 56%; P = .0005).[20,64] No benefit was noted in the arm that received standard balloon angioplasty with paclitaxel-containing contrast medium.[20]

The LEVANT 2 (Lutonix Paclitaxel-Coated Balloon for the Prevention of Femoropopliteal Restenosis) trial used a PCB with a concentration of 2 µg/mm² coated with polysorbate and sorbitol (n = 476).[65] Patients with Rutherford 2 to 5 symptoms and greater than 70% stenosis with a lesion length of less than 15 cm in the femoral or popliteal arteries were randomized in 2:1 fashion to Lutonix PCB (Bard Peripheral Vascular, Tempe, AZ) versus standard PTA. After predilation, patients who were anticipated to require stent placement (flow-limiting dissection or residual stenosis of >70%) were excluded from the study. Provisional stenting was performed less frequently following PCB (2.5% vs

6.9% PCB vs standard; P = .02). Primary patency (determined by duplex ultrasonography and/or TLR) at 12 months was higher in the PCB versus standard treatment group (65.2% vs 52.6%; P = .02).[65] The TLR rate was lower in the PCB arm, although it did not reach statistical significance (12.3% vs 16.8%, PCB vs standard balloon; P = .21).[65] Based on these data, the Lutonix Moxy Balloon was approved by the US FDA for patients with femoropopliteal disease.

The IN.PACT SFA (IN.PACT Admiral Drug-Coated Balloon vs Standard Balloon Angioplasty for the Treatment of Superficial Femoral Artery and Proximal Popliteal Artery) used the Admiral DCB (Medtronic Inc., Santa Rosa, CA) with a paclitaxel concentration of 3.5 µg/mm² coated with a urea excipient (n = 331).[66] This trial was composed of 2 phases, one in Europe and the second in the United States; there were minor variations in protocol between the 2 phases, including eligibility criteria, concomitant inflow, contralateral limb treatment, and predilation requirements. Patients enrolled had Rutherford 2 to 4 symptoms with 70% to 99% stenosis and lesion lengths 4 to 18 cm or occlusions with lengths of 10 cm or greater of the SFA or proximal popliteal artery. Randomization was in a 2:1 fashion to PCB versus standard PTA. At 12 months, freedom from restenosis defined by duplex-derived peak systolic velocity ratio of 2.4 or less or clinically driven TLR was higher in the PCB arm (82.2% vs 52.4%, PCB vs standard; P<.001).[66] At the 24-month follow-up, the primary patency rate remained higher in the PCB arm (78.9% vs 50.1%, PCB vs standard; P<.001), with clinically driven TLR rates that are significantly lower in the PCB arm (9.1% vs 28.1%, PCB vs standard; P<.001).[67] Based on these data, the IN.PACT Admiral DCB was approved by the US FDA for patients with femoropopliteal disease.

Data from the ILLUMENATE Pivotal IDE (Prospective, Randomized, Single-Blind, US Multi-Center Study to Evaluate Treatment of Obstructive Superficial Femoral Artery or Popliteal Lesions with a Novel Paclitaxel-Coated Percutaneous Angioplasty Balloon) trial using the newest DCB awaiting FDA approval, Stellarex (Spectranetics, Fremont, CA), was presented recently.[68] Stellarex uses a polyethylene glycol coating with a paclitaxel concentration of 2 µg/mm². The first-in-human, single-armed trial (n = 50) showed that the primary patency rate and freedom from clinically driven TLR were 89.5% and 90.0% at 12 months, and 80.3% and 85.8% at 24 months, respectively.[69] ILLUMENATE Global and Pivotal trials both seem to show promising results.[68,70] Specifically, in the US Pivotal data (n = 300, with 2:1 randomization to PCB) presented at TCT (transcatheter cardiovascular therapeutics), freedom from clinically driven TLR was better than PTA (93.6% vs 87.3%, PCB vs standard) at 12 months.[68,71] The final results on both of these trials have been presented but not yet published.

Below the Knee: Stent-Based Delivery

Given the differences in location and function, the infrapopliteal arteries (IPA) constitute an entirely distinct vascular bed compared with the SFA or coronary arteries. Although these vessels have the same nominal diameters as coronary arteries, they are not as muscular nor do they experience the same sort of pulsatile flow throughout the cardiac cycle. It is recognized that the incidence of ISR is higher and long-term benefit is lacking with revascularization of IPA,[1] such that revascularization should be reserved for those with concomitant inflow disease, to improve in-line flow, particularly in patients with CLI. Limited data exist for the use of DES in IPA. To date, 4 randomized controlled trials have compared the efficacy of coronary DES with BMS in IPA revascularization.[72–76] The trials recruited patients with symptomatic PAD with Rutherford 3 to 5 symptoms, but limited lesion lengths to less than 40 to 50 mm. All of the studies used coronary stents as the mode of DES, with 3 using the Cypher SES, and the DESTINY (Drug Eluting Stents in the Critically Ischemic Lower Leg) trial using Xience V (Abbott Vascular, Santa Clara, CA) EES.

Overall, the primary patency rate were all higher in the DES group compared with BMS group on follow-up. In the largest trial, YUKON-BTX (YUKON-drug-eluting Stent Below The Knee - Randomised Double-blind Study; n = 161), the 33-month target vessel revascularization for the entire population (combining CLI and severe claudication) was 9.2% versus 20% (SES vs BMS; P = .04).[74] In the second largest randomized controlled trial, DESTINY (n = 140), the 12-month primary patency rate was 85% versus 54% (EES vs BMS; P = .0001).[75] Similarly, in the ACHILLES (Comparing Angioplasty and DES in the Treatment of Subjects With Ischemic Infrapopliteal Arterial Disease) trial (n = 200), where the Cypher SES was compared with PTA, the clinically driven TLR was lower in the DES group at 1 year (10% vs 16.5%, SES vs PTA; P = .257). In comparison, the TLR rates of the same first-generation Cypher SES in the coronary arena was noted to be 7.8% at the 4-year follow-up,

approximately 4 times lower than the TLR of the same stent when deployed in the IPA.[77] Although primary patency and TLR seems to favor a DES over PTA or BMS in the IPA territory, these results are still sobering compared with that achieved in the coronary and SFA territories. For these reasons, stent placement in the IPA should be reserved for the stringently chosen patient with clinical necessity for stenting.

Below the Knee: Drug-Coated Balloons

An additional limitation of using DES in IPA lesions is the target lesion length. The majority of the aforementioned IPA trials limited the lesion length to less than 40 to 50 mm; although the ACHILLES trial allowed lesion lengths up to 120 mm, the mean lesion length was only 27 mm.[76] In reality, a high proportion of patients with IPA disease have long segment disease that would have precluded them from the DES trials. Furthermore, based on coronary data, it is known that increased length of stent implantation increases the risk of ISR.[78] This is likely to contribute to the ongoing unfavorable rates of TLR with DES in the IPA. DCBs in the IPA offer an alternative strategy of drug delivery without the additional commitment of long metallic stents.

The DEBATE-BTK (Drug-Eluting Balloon in Peripheral Intervention for Below the Knee Angioplasty Evaluation) trial was a randomized, single-center study that compared PCB with PTA in patients with diabetes mellitus, CLI with a Rutherford class of greater than 4, and significant stenosis or occlusion greater than 40 mm in at least 1 IPA vessel (n = 132).[79] The mean lesion length was approximately 130 mm, with a mean diameter stenosis of 97% in both arms. Patients underwent ultrasound duplex and angiography follow-up at 12 months. Restenosis of greater than 50% and clinically driven TLR were both more favorable in the PCB group (restenosis, 27% vs 74%, PCB vs PTA [P<.001]; TLR 18% vs 43%, DCB vs PTA [P = .002]).[79]

However, IN.PACT DEEP (Randomized Amphirion DEEP DEB v. Standard PTA for Treatment of Below the Knee Critical Limb Ischemia), a trial to investigate the use of IN.PACT Amphirion PCB in IPA revascularization for CLI patients did not show such favorable results (n = 358).[80] Despite randomization, there were significant differences between the 2 study groups: lesion length (101 mm vs 129 mm, PCB vs PTA; P = .002), concordant inflow disease (40.7% vs 28.8%, PCB vs PTA; P = .035), and prior target limb revascularization (32.2% vs 21.8%, PCB vs PTA; P = .047).[80] With these limitations in mind, neither the clinically driven TLR (9.2% vs 13.1%, PCB vs PTA; P = .291) nor late lumen loss were different between the 2 arms at 12 months of follow-up.[80]

The IDEAS (Infrapopliteal Drug-Eluting Angioplasty vs Stenting) trial was performed to directly compare the usefulness of PCB with DES in the IPA territory for patients with Rutherford stages 3 to 6 (n = 50).[81] The PCB used was IN.PACT Amphirion and DES were chosen based on department availability (included the Resolute [Medtronic, Santa Rosa, CA] zotarolimus-eluting stent, Cypher SES, and Promus EES [Boston Scientific, Marlborough, MA]). The mean lesion length differed, but was not statistically significant (148 mm vs 127 mm, DCB vs DES; P = .14).[81] Follow-up angiographic data were obtained at 12 months, which showed restenosis of greater than 50% to be greater in the PCB group (57.9% vs 28%; P = .0457) although the TLR was unaffected (13.6% vs 7.7%, PCB vs DES; P = .65).[81] This study is severely underpowered to draw any meaningful conclusions regarding the use of PCB compared with DES in IPA revascularization.

Although the use of DCB in the SFA offers promising outcomes as the technology for drug binding and delivery evolves,[82] the results in IPA revascularization are not as encouraging. The optimal technique for below-the-knee endovascular revascularization, particularly with long-segment stenoses, remains unclear at this point. Owing to the uncertainty and poor long-term patency rates, revascularization in this territory should be reserved for specific patients (eg, multilevel disease, poor outflow in the setting of CLI).

Atherectomy and Adjunctive Plaque Modification to Facilitate Peripheral Vascular Drug Delivery

There has been increasing interest in assessing the benefits of plaque modification and debulking before drug delivery, in an effort to the minimize barriers to drug absorption. Fanelli and colleagues[42] have shown that the length and degree of circumferential calcium can hinder the effects of DCB, with effects on primary patency, TLR, and late lumen loss (Fig. 9). With the increasing adoption of DCB in peripheral revascularization, the concept of using atherectomy and then antirestenotic therapy has garnered significant interest and clinical traction. To date, several studies have examined the hypothesis that removal of diffusion barriers will improve clinical efficacy of drug delivery.

The DEFINITIVE AR (Directional Atherectomy Followed by a Paclitaxel-Coated Balloon to Inhibit Restenosis and Maintain Vessel Patency) trial is a prospective, multicenter, randomized trial that evaluated the use of directional atherectomy (Turbohawk or Silverhawk [Medtronic, Santa Rosa, CA]) followed by PCB versus PCB alone for the treatment of de novo femoropopliteal stenosis (n = 102).[83] At the 1-year follow-up, primary patency by duplex ultrasonography and angiographic patency for long lesions (>100 mm) as well as severely calcified (dense, circumferential calcification extending for >50 mm) vessels were better in the directional atherectomy and antirestenotic therapy (DAART) group compared with PCB alone. Specifically for

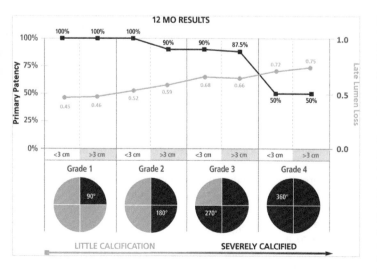

Fig. 9. Correlation exists between the severity of arterial calcification and both primary patency and late lumen loss at 12 months after angioplasty with the IN.PACT Admiral paclitaxel-coated balloon. The circumferential degree of calcium determines the grade (eg, grade 1, 0°–90°). Each grade is differentiated based on less than 3 cm or greater than 3 cm of calcium length. Primary patency was defined by freedom from restenosis by duplex peak systolic velocity ratio of less than 2.4 and target lesion revascularization. Late lumen loss was defined by the minimum lumen diameter (MLD) after the procedure minus the MLD at 12 months of follow-up. (Adapted from Fanelli F, Cannavale A, Gazzetti M, et al. Calcium burden assessment and impact on drug-eluting balloons in peripheral arterial disease. Cardiovasc Intervent Radiol 2014;37:898–907; and Zeller T. Setting a new benchmark: Eluvia clinical results and ongoing studies. Leipzig Interventional Course. Leipzig, Germany, January 26–27, 2016.)

duplex evaluation in the long lesion cohort, primary patency rates were 97% versus 86% (DAART vs PCB alone) and for the heavily calcified cohort, primary patency rates were 70% versus 63% (DAART vs PCB alone).[83] Although angiographic patency was also improved with DAART, this did not meet statistical significance. Two-year trial results have been presented but are not yet published.

Stavroulakis and colleagues[84] performed a single-arm study to evaluate the use of directional atherectomy (Turbohawk or Silverhawk) followed by PCB (IN.PACT Admiral) for popliteal artery lesions (n = 21). Primary patency rates were noted to be 95% and 90% at 12 and 18 months, respectively. Similarly, Cioppa and colleagues[85] performed DAART (Turbohawk followed by IN.PACT Admiral) on a small number of patients (n = 30) with either CLI or severe claudication found to have heavily calcified femoropopliteal arteries. Procedural success was 100% with a primary patency of 90%, clinically driven TLR rates of 10% at the 1-year follow-up.[85] Compared with prior studies, the need for bailout stenting (6.5%) and overall restenosis rates at 1 year were reduced.[85]

Conversely, there is a paucity of data for the application of DAART in IPA lesions. The ADCAT (Atherectomy and Drug-Coated Balloon Angioplasty in Treatment of Long Infrapopliteal Lesions) trial is a single-center, randomized study currently enrolling patients for the use of PCB with or without Turbohawk in de novo lesions in the IPA.

In addition to directional atherectomy, numerous devices exist for the removal of atheroma and calcification to facilitate vessel expansion and device delivery. Orbital atherectomy (Diamondback, Cardiovascular Systems, Inc, St. Paul, MN), rotational-aspirational atherectomy (JetStream, Boston Scientific, Marlborough, MA), and laser atherectomy (Excimer, Spectranetics, Fremont, CA) catheters are capable of providing various degrees of debulking. Preclinical animal model data using orbital atherectomy and adjunctive PCB therapy have shown that combination therapy seems to be safe in terms of vascular healing profile and drug tissue levels while decreasing plaque burden.[43] There are no head-to-head comparisons of these devices in the peripheral arteries, although their use is common and indications have considerable overlap.

As noted, the presence of ISR functions as a diffusion barrier for adequate drug delivery if a priori ablative therapy is not applied. Furthermore, compared with native atheroma, this tissue is at high risk of recoil. PTA with or without the use of scoring balloons has been unable to yield durable results (restenosis rates of 65%–73% at 6 months in 1 study).[86] An alternative mode of lesion modification is to use laser atherectomy to induce photochemical, photothermal, and photomechanical disruption of the fibrotic tissue. The EXCITE ISR (Excimer Laser Randomized Controlled Study for Treatment of Femoropopliteal In-Stent Restenosis) trial showed that patients with SFA ISR with Rutherford class 1 to 4 symptoms performed better with laser atherectomy and PTA compared with PTA alone (6-month freedom from TLR 73.5% vs 51.8% [P<.005]; total n = 250). When laser atherectomy is combined with DCB to treat ISR, the results are even more encouraging. Van Den Berg and colleagues[87] reported on a small series of 10 patients with SFA or popliteal ISR, treated with laser atherectomy followed by IN.PACT PCB. Over a mean follow-up of 7.6 months, there was no TLR and no evidence of neointimal hyperplasia on duplex and/or angiographic data (available on 7 of 10 patients).[87] Gandini and colleagues[88] subsequently reported on a small, single-center, randomized trial to evaluate the use of DCB with or without laser atherectomy in patients with CLI secondary to SFA chronic stent occlusion (n = 48). Patency rates were significantly better in the laser atherectomy cohort at 6 months (91.7% vs 58.3%, laser and DCB vs DCB only; P = .01) and at 12 months (66.7% vs 37.5%, laser and DCB vs DCB only; P = .01).[88] TLR (16.7% vs 50%, laser and DCB vs DCB only; P = .01) and limb salvage (91.7% vs 54.2%, laser and DCB vs DCB only; P = .003) were also in favor of laser atherectomy.[88]

Although there are a number of ongoing studies to evaluate the various atherectomy modalities in combination with DCB, there is a lack of formalized guidelines or appropriate use recommendations currently. At this time, it is reasonable to consider the adjunctive use of directional, rotational, laser, or orbital atherectomy devices in combination with DCB therapy, particularly for a patient with a heavily calcified and long lesion in the SFA. In the case of SFA ISR, laser atherectomy can be performed for tissue ablation followed by DCB in the hopes of curtailing the adverse, negative remodeling that lends to recalcitrant ISR. Significant clinical investigation in this area is expected in the coming years.

SUMMARY

Vascular drug delivery outside of the coronary arteries adheres to several first principles. Drug delivery is facilitated primarily by diffusion of solubilized drug from a stent or DCB coating deposited on the intimal surface of the target vessel. Specific and nonspecific binding along with well-described clearance mechanisms dictate steady-state arterial drug concentrations, which in turn direct clinical efficacy.

Extensive biochemical, mathematical, and engineering research in the last few decades has contributed tremendously to the improvement of our currently available DES for the coronary arteries. However, owing to the intrinsic differences between the coronary and peripheral vasculatures, the coronary technology cannot be translated directly into the peripheral domain. Future breakthroughs in peripheral vascular intervention that build on current drug delivery technologies will require investigators to acknowledge the similarities and differences between these vascular territories and capitalize on this knowledge to move the field forward.

REFERENCES

1. Gerhard-Herman MD, Gornik HL, Barrett C, et al. 2016 AHA/ACC guideline on the management of patients with lower extremity peripheral artery disease: a report of the American College of Cardiology/American Heart Association Task Force on clinical practice guidelines. J Am Coll Cardiol 2016. [Epub ahead of print].
2. Shishehbor MH, White CJ, Gray BH, et al. Critical limb ischemia: an expert statement. J Am Coll Cardiol 2016;68:2002–15.
3. Wilensky RL, March KL, Gradus-Pizlo I, et al. Vascular injury, repair, and restenosis after percutaneous transluminal angioplasty in the atherosclerotic rabbit. Circulation 1995;92:2995–3005.
4. Ponticos M, Smith BD. Extracellular matrix synthesis in vascular disease: hypertension, and atherosclerosis. J Biomed Res 2014;28:25–39.
5. Xu J, Shi G-P. Vascular wall extracellular matrix proteins and vascular diseases. Biochim Biophys Acta 2014;1842:2106–19.
6. Wagenseil JE, Mecham RP. Vascular extracellular matrix and arterial mechanics. Physiol Rev 2009; 89:957–89.
7. Hwang C-W, Edelman ER. Arterial ultrastructure influences transport of locally delivered drugs. Circ Res 2002;90:826–32.
8. Byrne RA, Joner M, Kastrati A. Stent thrombosis and restenosis: what have we learned and where are we going? The Andreas Grüntzig Lecture ESC 2014. Eur Heart J 2015;36:3320–31.
9. Ako J, Bonneau HN, Honda Y, et al. Design criteria for the ideal drug-eluting stent. Am J Cardiol 2007; 100:S3–9.
10. Indolfi C, De Rosa S, Colombo A. Bioresorbable vascular scaffolds - basic concepts and clinical outcome. Nat Rev Cardiol 2016;13(12):719–29.
11. Serruys PW, Chevalier B, Sotomi Y, et al. Comparison of an everolimus-eluting bioresorbable scaffold with an everolimus-eluting metallic stent for the treatment of coronary artery stenosis (ABSORB II): a 3 year, randomised, controlled, single-blind, multicentre clinical trial. Lancet 2016;388(10059):2479–91.
12. Hou D, Huibregtse BA, Eppihimer M, et al. Fluorocopolymer-coated nitinol self-expanding paclitaxel-eluting stent: pharmacokinetics and vascular biology responses in a porcine iliofemoral model. EuroIntervention 2016;12:790–7.
13. McGinty S, Pontrelli G. A general model of coupled drug release and tissue absorption for drug delivery devices. J Control Release 2015;217:327–36.
14. Lovich MA, Edelman ER. Mechanisms of transmural heparin transport in the rat abdominal aorta after local vascular delivery. Circ Res 1995;77:1143–50.
15. Elmalak O, Lovich MA, Edelman E. Correlation of transarterial transport of various dextrans with their physicochemical properties. Biomaterials 2000;21: 2263–72.
16. Smith EJ, Rothman MT. Antiproliferative coatings for the treatment of coronary heart disease. J Interv Cardiol 2003;16:475–83.
17. Tzafriri AR, Edelman ER. Endovascular drug delivery and drug elution systems. Interv Cardiol Clin 2016;5:307–20.
18. Daemen J, Serruys PW. Drug-eluting stent update 2007. Part I: a survey of current and future generation drug-eluting stents: meaningful advances or more of the same? Circulation 2007;116:316–28.
19. Frenning G. Modelling drug release from inert matrix systems: from moving-boundary to continuous-field descriptions. Int J Pharm 2011;418:88–99.
20. Tepe G, Zeller T, Albrecht T, et al. Local delivery of paclitaxel to inhibit restenosis during angioplasty of the leg. N Engl J Med 2008;358:689–99.
21. Scheller B, Speck U, Schmitt A, et al. Addition of paclitaxel to contrast media prevents restenosis after coronary stent implantation. J Am Coll Cardiol 2003;42:1415–20.
22. Scheller B, Speck U, Romeike B, et al. Contrast media as carriers for local drug delivery. Successful inhibition of neointimal proliferation in the porcine coronary stent model. Eur Heart J 2003; 24:1462–7.
23. Scheller B, Speck U, Abramjuk C, et al. Paclitaxel balloon coating, a novel method for prevention and therapy of restenosis. Circulation 2004;110: 810–4.
24. Albrecht T, Speck U, Baier C, et al. Reduction of stenosis due to intimal hyperplasia after stent supported angioplasty of peripheral arteries by local administration of paclitaxel in swine. Invest Radiol 2007;42:579–85.
25. Speck U, Cremers B, Kelsch B, et al. Do pharmacokinetics explain persistent restenosis inhibition by a

single dose of paclitaxel? Circ Cardiovasc Interv 2012;5:392–400.

26. Radke PW, Joner M, Joost A, et al. Vascular effects of paclitaxel following drug-eluting balloon angioplasty in a porcine coronary model: the importance of excipients. EuroIntervention 2011;7:730–7.

27. Gray WA, Granada JF. Drug-coated balloons for the prevention of vascular restenosis. Circulation 2010;121:2672–80.

28. Tzafriri AR, Vukmirovic N, Kolachalama VB, et al. Lesion complexity determines arterial drug distribution after local drug delivery. J Control Release 2010;142:332–8.

29. Wan WK, Lovich MA, Hwang CW, et al. Measurement of drug distribution in vascular tissue using quantitative fluorescence microscopy. J Pharm Sci 1999;88:822–9.

30. Goriely AR, Baldwin AL, Secomb TW. Transient diffusion of albumin in aortic walls: effects of binding to medial elastin layers. Am J Physiol Heart Circ Physiol 2007;292:H2195–201.

31. Sirianni RW, Kremer J, Guler I, et al. Effect of extracellular matrix elements on the transport of paclitaxel through an arterial wall tissue mimic. Biomacromolecules 2008;9:2792–8.

32. Balakrishnan B, Dooley J, Kopia G, et al. Thrombus causes fluctuations in arterial drug delivery from intravascular stents. J Control Release 2008;131: 173–80.

33. Alfonso F, Byrne RA, Rivero F, et al. Current treatment of in-stent restenosis. J Am Coll Cardiol 2014;63:2659–73.

34. Creel CJ, Lovich MA, Edelman ER. Arterial paclitaxel distribution and deposition. Circ Res 2000; 86:879–84.

35. Lovich MA, Philbrook M, Sawyer S, et al. Arterial heparin deposition: role of diffusion, convection, and extravascular space. Am J Physiol 1998;275: H2236–42.

36. Tzafriri AR, Groothuis A, Price GS, et al. Stent elution rate determines drug deposition and receptor-mediated effects. J Control Release 2012;161:918–26.

37. Tzafriri AR, Lerner EI, Flashner-Barak M, et al. Mathematical modeling and optimization of drug delivery from intratumorally injected microspheres. Clin Cancer Res 2005;11:826–34.

38. Artzi N, Tzafriri AR, Faucher KM, et al. Sustained efficacy and arterial drug retention by a fast drug eluting cross-linked fatty acid coronary stent coating. Ann Biomed Eng 2016;44:276–86.

39. Kolachalama VB, Pacetti SD, Franses JW, et al. Mechanisms of tissue uptake and retention in zotarolimus-coated balloon therapy. Circulation 2013;127:2047–55.

40. McGinty S, Pontrelli G. On the role of specific drug binding in modelling arterial eluting stents. J Math Chem 2016;54:967–76.

41. Mandal PK, Sarifuddin, Kolachalama VB. Computational model of drug-coated balloon delivery in a patient-specific arterial vessel with heterogeneous tissue composition. Cardiovasc Eng Technol 2016; 7(4):406–19.

42. Fanelli F, Cannavale A, Gazzetti M, et al. Calcium burden assessment and impact on drug-eluting balloons in peripheral arterial disease. Cardiovasc Intervent Radiol 2014;37:898–907.

43. Tellez A, Dattilo R, Mustapha JA, et al. Biological effect of orbital atherectomy and adjunctive paclitaxel-coated balloon therapy on vascular healing and drug retention: early experimental insights into the familial hypercholesterolaemic swine model of femoral artery stenosis. EuroIntervention 2014;10:1002–8.

44. Buszman PP, Tellez A, Afari ME, et al. Tissue uptake, distribution, and healing response after delivery of paclitaxel via second-generation iopromide-based balloon coating: a comparison with the first-generation technology in the iliofemoral porcine model. JACC Cardiovasc Interv 2013;6:883–90.

45. Granada JF, Stenoien M, Buszman PP, et al. Mechanisms of tissue uptake and retention of paclitaxel-coated balloons: impact on neointimal proliferation and healing. Open Heart 2014;1:e000117.

46. Granada JF. "Technical and biologic challenges for future DCB development". 2nd International DEB Symposium. Berlin, Germany, November 16–17, 2012.

47. Buszman PP, Milewski K, Żurakowski A, et al. Experimental evaluation of pharmacokinetic profile and biological effect of a novel paclitaxel microcrystalline balloon coating in the iliofemoral territory of swine. Catheter Cardiovasc Interv 2014;83:325–33.

48. Duda SH, Pusich B, Richter G, et al. Sirolimus-eluting stents for the treatment of obstructive superficial femoral artery disease: six-month results. Circulation 2002;106:1505–9.

49. Duda SH, Bosiers M, Lammer J, et al. Sirolimus-eluting versus bare nitinol stent for obstructive superficial femoral artery disease: the SIROCCO II trial. J Vasc Interv Radiol 2005;16:331–8.

50. Duda SH, Bosiers M, Lammer J, et al. Drug-eluting and bare nitinol stents for the treatment of atherosclerotic lesions in the superficial femoral artery: long-term results from the SIROCCO trial. J Endovasc Ther 2006;13:701–10.

51. Lammer J, Bosiers M, Zeller T, et al. First clinical trial of nitinol self-expanding everolimus-eluting stent implantation for peripheral arterial occlusive disease. J Vasc Surg 2011;54:394–401.

52. Litsky J, Chanda A, Stilp E, et al. Critical evaluation of stents in the peripheral arterial disease of the superficial femoral artery – focus on the paclitaxel eluting stent. Med Devices (Auckl) 2014;7:149–56.

53. Schillinger M, Sabeti S, Loewe C, et al. Balloon angioplasty versus implantation of nitinol stents in the

superficial femoral artery. N Engl J Med 2006;354: 1879–88.

54. Dake MD, Ansel GM, Jaff MR, et al. Paclitaxel-eluting stents show superiority to balloon angioplasty and bare metal stents in femoropopliteal disease: twelve-month Zilver PTX randomized study results. Circ Cardiovasc Interv 2011;4:495–504.

55. Dake MD, Ansel GM, Jaff MR, et al. Sustained safety and effectiveness of paclitaxel-eluting stents for femoropopliteal lesions: 2-year follow-up from the zilver PTX randomized and single-arm clinical studies. J Am Coll Cardiol 2013;61:2417–27.

56. Dake MD, Ansel GM, Jaff MR, et al. Durable clinical effectiveness with paclitaxel-eluting stents in the femoropopliteal artery: 5-year results of the zilver PTX randomized trial. Circulation 2016;133:1472–83 [discussion: 1483].

57. Muller-Hulsbeck S, Keirse K, Zeller T, et al. Twelve-month results from the MAJESTIC trial of the Eluvia paclitaxel-eluting stent for treatment of obstructive femoropopliteal disease. J Endovasc Ther 2016;23: 701–7.

58. Zeller T. Setting a new benchmark: Eluvia clinical results and ongoing studies. Leipzig Interventional Course; Leipzig, Germany, January 26–27, 2016.

59. Scheinert D. The latest treatment approach and current developments in SFA. Leipzig Interventional Course; Leipzig, Germany, January 26–27, 2016.

60. Dake MD, Van Alstine WG, Zhou Q, et al. Polymer-free paclitaxel-coated zilver PTX Stents–evaluation of pharmacokinetics and comparative safety in porcine arteries. J Vasc Interv Radiol 2011;22: 603–10.

61. Peeters P, Bosiers M, Verbist J, et al. Preliminary results after application of absorbable metal stents in patients with critical limb ischemia. J Endovasc Ther 2005;12:1–5.

62. Varcoe RL, Schouten O, Thomas SD, et al. Initial experience with the absorb bioresorbable vascular scaffold below the knee: six-month clinical and imaging outcomes. J Endovasc Ther 2015;22:226–32.

63. Lammer J, Bosiers M, Deloose K, et al. Bioresorbable everolimus-eluting vascular scaffold for patients with peripheral artery disease (ESPRIT I): 2-year clinical and imaging results. JACC Cardiovasc Interv 2016;9:1178–87.

64. Tepe G, Schnorr B, Albrecht T, et al. Angioplasty of femoral-popliteal arteries with drug-coated balloons5-year follow-up of the THUNDER trial. JACC Cardiovasc Interv 2015;8:102–8.

65. Rosenfield K, Jaff MR, White CJ, et al. Trial of a paclitaxel-coated balloon for femoropopliteal artery disease. N Engl J Med 2015;373:145–53.

66. Tepe G, Laird J, Schneider P, et al. Drug-coated balloon versus standard percutaneous transluminal angioplasty for the treatment of superficial femoral and popliteal peripheral artery disease: 12-month results from the IN.PACT SFA randomized trial. Circulation 2015;131:495–502.

67. Laird JR, Schneider PA, Tepe G, et al. Durability of treatment effect using a drug-coated balloon for femoropopliteal lesions24-month results of IN.PACT SFA. J Am Coll Cardiol 2015;66:2329–38.

68. McKeown LA. ILLUMENATE: low-dose DCB bests angioplasty alone in complex patients with SFA/popliteal lesions. TCTMD; Washington, DC, October 29–November 2, 2016.

69. Schroeder H, Meyer D-R, Lux B, et al. Two-year results of a low-dose drug-coated balloon for revascularization of the femoropopliteal artery: outcomes from the ILLUMENATE first-in-human study. Catheter Cardiovasc Interv 2015;86:278–86.

70. Spectranetics. 12-month interim ILLUMENATE Global study data presented on Spectranetics' Stellarex drug-coated balloon at Charing Cross. 2016. Availaible at: http://investor.spectranetics.com/phoenix.zhtml?c=71603&p=irol-newsArticle&ID=2161310.

71. Lyden SP. ILLUMENATE US: a prospective, randomized trial of a paclitaxel-coated balloon vs an uncoated balloon for treatment of diseased superficial femoral and popliteal arteries. TCT; Washington, DC, October 29–November 2, 2016.

72. Falkowski A, Poncyljusz W, Wilk G, et al. The evaluation of primary stenting of sirolimus-eluting versus bare-metal stents in the treatment of atherosclerotic lesions of crural arteries. Eur Radiol 2009;19: 966–74.

73. Tepe G, Schmehl J, Heller S, et al. Drug eluting stents versus PTA with GP IIb/IIIa blockade below the knee in patients with current ulcers–the BELOW Study. J Cardiovasc Surg (Torino) 2010; 51:203–12.

74. Rastan A, Brechtel K, Krankenberg H, et al. Sirolimus-eluting stents for treatment of infrapopliteal arteries reduce clinical event rate compared to bare-metal stents: long-term results from a randomized trial. J Am Coll Cardiol 2012;60:587–91.

75. Bosiers M, Scheinert D, Peeters P, et al. Randomized comparison of everolimus-eluting versus bare-metal stents in patients with critical limb ischemia and infrapopliteal arterial occlusive disease. J Vasc Surg 2012;55:390–8.

76. Scheinert D, Katsanos K, Zeller T, et al. A prospective randomized multicenter comparison of balloon angioplasty and infrapopliteal stenting with the sirolimus-eluting stent in patients with ischemic peripheral arterial disease: 1-year results from the ACHILLES trial. J Am Coll Cardiol 2012; 60:2290–5.

77. Stone GW, Moses JW, Ellis SG, et al. Safety and efficacy of sirolimus- and paclitaxel-eluting coronary stents. N Engl J Med 2007;356:998–1008.

78. Dangas GD, Claessen BE, Caixeta A, et al. In-Stent Restenosis in the Drug-Eluting Stent Era. J Am Coll Cardiol 2010;56:1897–907.

79. Liistro F, Porto I, Angioli P, et al. Drug-eluting balloon in peripheral intervention for below the knee angioplasty evaluation (DEBATE-BTK): a randomized trial in diabetic patients with critical limb ischemia. Circulation 2013;128(6):615–21.

80. Zeller T, Baumgartner I, Scheinert D, et al. Drug-eluting balloon versus standard balloon angioplasty for infrapopliteal arterial revascularization in critical limb ischemia12-month results from the IN.PACT DEEP randomized trial. J Am Coll Cardiol 2014;64:1568–76.

81. Siablis D, Kitrou PM, Spiliopoulos S, et al. Paclitaxel-coated balloon angioplasty versus drug-eluting stenting for the treatment of infrapopliteal long-segment arterial occlusive disease the IDEAS randomized controlled trial. JACC Cardiovasc Interv 2014;7:1048–56.

82. Kayssi A, Al-Atassi T, Oreopoulos G, et al. Drug-eluting balloon angioplasty versus uncoated balloon angioplasty for peripheral arterial disease of the lower limbs. Cochrane Database Syst Rev 2016;(8):CD011319.

83. Zeller T. When DCB is not enough: is there a need for a new DAART study? Leipzig Interventional Course; Leipzig, Germany, January 26–27, 2016.

84. Stavroulakis K, Bisdas T, Torsello G, et al. Combined directional atherectomy and drug-eluting balloon angioplasty for isolated popliteal artery lesions in patients with peripheral artery disease. J Endovasc Ther 2015;22:847–52.

85. Cioppa A, Stabile E, Popusoi G, et al. Combined treatment of heavy calcified femoro-popliteal lesions using directional atherectomy and a paclitaxel coated balloon: one-year single centre clinical results. Cardiovasc Revasc Med 2012;13:219–23.

86. Dick P, Sabeti S, Mlekusch W, et al. Conventional balloon angioplasty versus peripheral cutting balloon angioplasty for treatment of femoropopliteal artery in-stent restenosis: initial experience. Radiology 2008;248:297–302.

87. Van Den Berg JC, Pedrotti M, Canevascini R, et al. Endovascular treatment of in-stent restenosis using excimer laser angioplasty and drug eluting balloons. J Cardiovasc Surg (Torino) 2012;53:215–22.

88. Gandini R, Del Giudice C, Merolla S, et al. Treatment of chronic SFA in-stent occlusion with combined laser atherectomy and drug-eluting balloon angioplasty in patients with critical limb ischemia: a single-center, prospective, randomized study. J Endovasc Ther 2013;20:805–14.

Drug-Coated Balloons
Current Outcomes and Future Directions

CrossMark

Ananya Kondapalli, MD[a], Barbara A. Danek, MD[b],
Houman Khalili, MD[a,b],
Haekyung Jeon-Slaughter, PhD[a,b],
Subhash Banerjee, MD[a,b],*

KEYWORDS

- Drug-coated balloons • Paclitaxel • Endovascular intervention
- Femoropopliteal peripheral artery • Infrapopliteal peripheral artery

KEY POINTS

- Although outcomes with DCB in the femoropopliteal region are promising, the ideal treatment strategy for lesions in the infrapopliteal arterial distribution remains an unmet need.
- The ideal antiplatelet regimen after peripheral arterial interventions, including DCB, has not been adequately defined.
- Future iterations of the DCB will likely include improved drug formulations, allowing for greater efficacy and limiting systemic toxic effects.
- The importance of specific excipients is being explored.
- Cost-based analyses of treatment strategies explore an increasingly important aspect of medical care, and will no doubt factor into the future of drug-coated balloons.

INTRODUCTION

Endovascular intervention is the first-line therapy for peripheral artery disease (PAD) and is associated with decreased morbidity and mortality compared with surgical interventions.[1] The main disadvantage to percutaneous transluminal angioplasty (PTA) and stenting continues to be the high rates of in-stent restenosis and stent fracture that can affect long-term clinical outcomes.[2,3] Neointimal proliferation and restenosis occur in more than 60% of patients treated with PTA for PAD.[4] Use of drug-eluting stents (DES) to prevent restenosis has displayed varying results. Sirolimus-eluting stents show no difference in outcomes compared with bare metal stents (BMS),[5] but paclitaxel-eluting stents have improved outcomes and decreased rates of restenosis.[6] Paclitaxel may be more effective in preventing restenosis in peripheral arteries because of their high proportion of extracellular matrix compared with coronary arteries, leading to better drug penetration and retention with hydrophobic drugs, such as paclitaxel.

Paclitaxel is an antiproliferative agent that inhibits neointimal proliferation even at low doses.

Financial Disclosure: Drs A. Kondapolli, B.A. Danek, H. Khalili, and H. Jeon-Slaughter have no relevant conflict of interest to disclose. Dr S. Banerjee has received research grants from Boston Scientific and Medicines Company; consultant/speaker honoraria from Gilead, St Jude, Cordis, Boehinger Ingerheim, Sanofi, and Medtronic; and reports ownership of Mdcare Global (spouse) and intellectual property of HygeiaTel.
Role of the Funding Source: The current study received no financial support for preparation of the article.
^a Division of Cardiology, Department of Medicine, University of Texas Southwestern Medical Center, 4500 South Lancaster Road (111a), Dallas, TX 75216, USA; ^b Division of Cardiology, Department of Medicine, Veterans Affairs North Texas Health Care System, 4500 South Lancaster Road (111a), Dallas, TX 75216, USA
* Corresponding author. 4500 South Lancaster Road (111a), Dallas, TX 75216.
E-mail address: subhash.banerjee@utsouthwestern.edu

Inhibition of neointimal proliferation leads to decreased rates of restenosis.[7,8] More recently, paclitaxel has been used as the drug of choice on drug-coated balloons (DCB). The advantage of using paclitaxel-coated balloons is the ability to deliver the necessary drug to the affected areas without a permanent vascular prosthesis. This article provides an overview of the clinical evidence for paclitaxel-coated balloons in the femoropopliteal and infrapopliteal peripheral artery distributions and future directions in this area.

TRIALS COMPARING DRUG-COATED BALLOONS WITH STANDARD PERCUTANEOUS TRANSLUMINAL ANGIOPLASTY IN FEMOROPOPLITEAL LESIONS

The earliest trials comparing DCB with PTA for the treatment of femoropopliteal lesions are the FemPac (Paclitaxel-Coated versus Uncoated Balloon: Femoral Paclitaxel Randomized Pilot Trial), THUNDER (Local Taxane with Short Exposure for Reduction of Restenosis in Distal Arteries), LEVANT I (Lutonix Paclitaxel-Coated Balloon for the Prevention of Femoropopliteal Restenosis), and PACIFIER (Paclitaxel-coated Balloons in Femoral Indication to Defeat Restenosis) trials. These were all randomized controlled trials with a primary end point of 6-month late lumen loss (LLL) defined as the difference between minimum luminal diameter after the procedure and at 6-month follow-up.[9–12] A study performed by Mauri and colleagues[13] demonstrated that LLL was the most sensitive marker for identifying restenosis because of neointimal proliferation. In each of these trials the DCB group was associated with significantly reduced LLL compared with the PTA group. Secondary outcomes including target lesion revascularization (TLR) were also significantly lower in the DCB group compared with PTA. Although these trials demonstrate the efficacy of DCB in treating femoropopliteal lesions, they do not provide information about long-term outcomes.

Micari and colleagues[14] examined 2-year outcomes after treatment with paclitaxel-coated balloons. The primary end point was primary patency rate defined as the absence of TLR, occlusions, or greater than or equal to 50% stenosis in the target lesions 24 months after treatment. Patients had a high primary patency rate (71%) and were observed to have significant improvements in ankle-brachial index and Rutherford class 2 years after treatment with DCB. The mean lesion length in the previously mentioned studies was 70 to 80 mm, with total occlusions representing less than 30% of the lesions. The DEBATE-SFA (Drug-Eluting Balloon in Peripheral Intervention for the Superficial Femoral Artery) trial compared treatment with DCB before insertion of a BMS with standard PTA before BMS in complex superficial femoral artery lesions.[15] Patients in the DEBATE-SFA trial had longer lesion lengths (>90 mm) and more than 50% of the lesions in the DCB group and 60% of the lesions in the PTA group were total occlusions. Patients in the DCB group had significantly lower rates of binary restenosis, defined as greater than or equal to 50% stenosis in the target lesion, 12 months after the procedure (17% vs 47%; $P = .008$). The use of nitinol self-expanding stents and inclusion of longer and more occluded lesions differentiates the DEBATE-SFA trial from previous trials in this area. Additionally, 69% of patients in the PTA group and 79% of patients in the DCB group had critical limb ischemia (CLI) in this trial compared with less than 10% of patients in previous trials.

The LEVANT 2 (Moxy Drug Coated Balloon versus Standard Balloon Angioplasty for the Treatment of Femoropopliteal Arteries) trial found higher primary patency rates in the DCB group compared with PTA in a study with a much larger sample size (n = 476). However, unlike the previous smaller randomized control trials, there was no significant difference in TLR between the two groups. This may be caused by several factors including the lower rate of TLR observed in the PTA group in this study compared with previous studies and exclusion of patients requiring stent placement.[16]

The findings from the IN.PACT SFA (Randomized Trial of IN.PACT Admiral Drug-Eluting Balloon versus Standard Percutaneous Transluminal Angioplasty for the Treatment of SFA and Proximal Popliteal Arterial Disease) trial support the earlier data showing higher primary patency rates and lower TLR with DCBs; however, there was a higher 24-month all-cause mortality rate in the DCB group. The mortality rate in the DCB group was 8.1%, which is in the range for the overall mortality rate for patients with PAD.[2] Three-year follow-up of IN.PACT SFA has confirmed superior patency and TLR with DCB, with no difference in the incidence of major adverse cardiovascular events. Higher all-cause mortality in the DCB group has persisted at 3 years, but these deaths occurred at a median of 1.8 years, and they were mostly unrelated to the procedure.[17] The FAIR (Femoral Artery In-Stent Restenosis) trial was the first to compare DCB with standard balloon angioplasty for treatment of SFA in-stent restenosis and reported that use of paclitaxel-coated balloons significantly reduced recurrent restenosis at 1 year.[18]

Newer trials for femoropopliteal lesions are shifting focus to testing the efficacy of specific devices, different formulations, and varying doses of paclitaxel. The BIOLUX P-I (BIOLUX P-I First-In-Man Study) trial targeted the efficacy of a specific DCB that had not been used in prior studies.[19] This trial used a different drug formulation with the excipient butyryl-tri-hexyl-citrate, which is intended to improve uptake of paclitaxel by the arterial wall. The formula was found to be effective in coronary artery disease, but has not been studied in PAD. The ILLUMENATE first-in-human trial used a smaller dose of paclitaxel (2 $\mu g/mm^2$) compared with previous studies (3 $\mu g/mm^2$), limiting the possibility of systemic impact of the drug.[20] The DCB groups in both trials had significantly decreased LLL compared with standard PTA.

The most recently published trial on DCB in the femoropopliteal region, the SFA-Long (Drug Eluting Balloon and Long Lesions of Superficial Femoral Artery Ischemic Vascular Disease) trial, examined more complex lesions with a mean length of 251 mm (longest to date) and 49.5% total occlusions. Similar to previous trials, treatment with paclitaxel-coated balloons resulted in high primary patency rates at 1 year.[21] The newest data for femoropopliteal lesions is from the ILLUMENATE Pivotal trial, which compared Stellarex DCB with PTA.[22] This trial's patient population was noted to be the most complex patient population studied thus far and includes a large percentage of patients with severe calcification (43.9%), diabetes mellitus (49.5%), renal insufficiency (18%), and cardiovascular disease (45%). The DCB group had higher primary patency and increased freedom from TLR at 12 months.

In summary, DCBs have been established as superior to PTA for the treatment of lesions in the femoropopliteal region, with ongoing optimization for further improved outcomes (Table 1).[9–12,14–16,18,19,21–28]

TRIALS COMPARING DRUG-COATED BALLOONS WITH STANDARD PERCUTANEOUS TRANSLUMINAL ANGIOPLASTY IN INFRAPOPLITEAL LESIONS

Before discussing the current outcomes studies that evaluated DCB efficacy in infrapopliteal lesions, it is important to note some key differences between the femoropopliteal and infrapopliteal lesions studied in the major trials and reports.

These differences include longer lesion lengths, smaller vessel diameter, higher percentage of patients with CLI, and higher percentage of total occlusions in the infrapopliteal lesions. Patients were consistently found to have Rutherford category 5 lesions in the infrapopliteal arteries compared with Rutherford category 3 in most of the femoropopliteal artery trials excluding the DEBATE-SFA trial. The infrapopliteal lesions were more than 100 mm in length compared with the femoropopliteal lesions, which were approximately 70 mm or less.

Schmidt and colleagues[24] studied the rate of binary restenosis in infrapopliteal lesions treated with DCB and found the restenosis rate to be significantly reduced compared with uncoated balloons; however, the patients were followed up only 3 months after the procedure. The DEBATE-BTK (Drug-Eluting Balloon in Peripheral Intervention for Below the Knee Angioplasty Evaluation) trial was a randomized control trial that studied 1-year restenosis rates after treatment with DCB specifically in patients with diabetes and concomitant CLI. Patients treated with the DCB had a significantly decreased restenosis rate, TLR, and occlusions at 1 year follow-up.[25] The IN.PACT DEEP (Randomized Study of IN.PACT Amphirion Drug Eluting Balloon versus Standard PTA for the Treatment of Below the Knee Critical Limb Ischemia) trial was performed to confirm the findings of the study by Schmidt and colleagues[24] and the single-center randomized DEBATE-BTK trial.[25] This multicenter randomized controlled trial showed no statistically significant difference in LLL or TLR rates between the DCB and PTA groups. Additionally, the rate of major amputation was higher in the DCB group compared with the PTA group (8.8% vs 3.6%; $P = .08$).[26]

After promising results using the Passeo-18 Lux device in femoropopliteal lesions, the BIOLUX P-II (BIOTRONIK'S First-in-Human Study of the Passeo-18 LUX Drug-Releasing PTA Balloon Catheter versus the Uncoated Passeo-18 PTA Balloon Catheter in Subjects Requiring Revascularization of Infrapopliteal Arteries) trial prospectively compared this DCB device with conventional PTA in infrapopliteal lesions. The primary end point of 6-month primary patency loss was not significantly different in the DCB group compared with the PTA group. Both the DCB and PTA groups had good outcomes in the trial and although this shows that the Passeo-18 LUX device is safe to use for infrapopliteal occlusions, it does not demonstrate superiority of treating infrapopliteal lesions with a DCB compared with standard PTA.[27]

Table 1
Published studies of paclitaxel-coated balloons

First Author, Year	Trial Name	N	DCB Model, n	Formulation, Dose	Control, n	1° Endpoint	1° Outcome
Above the knee							
Tepe et al,[9] 2008	THUNDER	154	PTA coated with paclitaxel, 48	Paclitaxel-iopromide, 3.0	PTA, 54; PTA + PIC, 52	6 mo LLL	0.4 ± 1.2 vs PTA 1.7 ± 1.8 vs PIC 2.2 ± 1.6 mm (P<.001)
Werk et al,[10] 2008	FemPac	87	PTA coated with paclitaxel, 45	Paclitaxel-iopromide, 3.0	PTA, 42	6 mo LLL	0.5 ± 1.1 vs 1.0 ± 1.1 mm (P = .031)
Scheinert et al,[11] 2014	LEVANT I	101	Lutonix DCB Moxy, 49	Paclitaxel-polysorbate/sorbitol, 2.0	PTA, 52	6 mo LLL	0.46 ± 1.13 vs 1.09 ± 1.07 mm (P = .016)
Werk et al,[12] 2012	PACIFIER	91	IN.PACT Pacific, 44	FreePac Paclitaxel-urea, 3.0	PTA, 47	6 mo LLL	−0.01 (95% CI, −0.29 to 0.26) vs 0.65 (95% CI 0.37 to −0.93) mm (P = .001)
Micari et al,[14] 2013	—	105	IN.PACT Admiral, 105	Paclitaxel-urea, 3.0	N/A	12 mo PP	72.4% (P<.001)
Liistro et al,[15] 2013	DEBATE-SFA	104	IN.PACT Admiral + BMS, 53	Paclitaxel-urea, 3.0	PTA + BMS, 51	12 mo BRS	17% vs 47% (P = .008)
Rosenfield et al,[16] 2015	LEVANT II	476	Lutonix DCB Moxy, 316	Paclitaxel-polysorbate/sorbitol, 2.0	PTA, 160	12 mo PP	65.2% vs 52.6% (P = .02)
Tepe et al,[23] 2015	IN.PACT SFA II	331	IN.PACT Admiral, 220	Paclitaxel-urea, 3.0	PTA, 111	12 mo PP	82.2% vs 52.4% (P<.001)
Krankenberg et al,[18] 2015	FAIR	119	IN.PACT, 62	Paclitaxel-urea, 3.0	PTA, 57	6 mo BRS	15.4% vs 44.7% (P = .002)
Scheinert et al,[19] 2015	BIOLUX P-I	60	Passeo-18 Lux, 30	Paclitaxel-BTHC, 3.0	PTA, 30	6 mo LLL	0.51 ± 0.72 vs 1.04 ± 1.00 mm, P = .033
Schroeder et al,[20] 2015	ILLUMENATE FIH	50	Stellarex DCB, 50	Paclitaxel-Polyethylene glycol,2.0	N/A	12 mo PP	89.5%
Lyden,[22] 2016	ILLUMENATE Pivotal	300	Stellarex DCB	Paclitaxel, 2.0	PTA	12 mo PP; 12 mo freedom from TLR	PP: 82.3% vs 70.9% Freedom from TLR: 93.6% vs 87.3%
Micari et al,[21] 2016	SFA-LONG	105	IN.PACT Admiral, 105	Paclitaxel-urea, 3.0	N/A	12 mo PP	83.2%

Below the knee							
Schmidt et al,[24] 2011	—	104	IN.PACT Amphirion, 104	Paclitaxel-urea, 3.0	N/A	3 mo BRS	27.4%
Liistro et al,[25] 2013	DEBATE-BTK	132	IN.PACT Amphirion, 65	Paclitaxel-urea, 3.0	PTA, 67	12 mo BRS	27% vs 74% (P<.001)
Zeller et al,[26] 2014	IN.PACT DEEP	358	IN.PACT Amphirion, 239	Paclitaxel-urea, 3.0	PTA, 119	12 mo TLR 12 mo LLL	TLR: 9.2% vs 13.1% (P = .29); LLL: 0.61 ± 0.78 vs 0.62 ± 0.78 mm (P = .95)
Zeller et al,[27] 2015	BIOLUX P-II	72	Passeo-18 Lux, 36	Paclitaxel-BTHC, 3.0	PTA, 36	1 mo MAE[a] 6 mo PL	MAE: 0% vs 8.3% (P = .24); PL: 17.1% vs 26.1% (P = .30)
Siablis et al,[28] 2014	IDEAS I	50	Paclitaxel, 25	N/A	DES, 25	6 mo BRS	57.9% vs 28.0% (P = .048)
Steiner et al,[29] 2016	—	248	Lutonix DCB Moxy, 248	Paclitaxel-polysorbate/ sorbitol, 2.0	N/A	9 mo TLR	15.9%

Abbreviations: BRS, binary restenosis; BTHC, butyryl-tri-hexyl-citrate; CI, confidence interval; FIH, first-in-human; MAE, major adverse event rate; PIC, paclitaxel in contrast; PL, patency loss; PP, primary patency; TCT, transcatheter cardiovascular therapeutics.
[a] Defined as death, major amputation of target extremity, target lesion thrombosis, TLR, and target vessel revascularization.

Results from the IDEAS (Infrapopliteal Drug Eluting Angioplasty versus Stenting for the Treatment of Long-Segment Artery Disease) trial, which compared DCB with DES (either Resolute [Medtronic, Brescia, Italy], Cypher [Cordis, Bridgewater, NJ], or Promus [Boston Scientific, Natick, MA] according to availability) in infrapopliteal arteries, demonstrated decreased restenosis in the DES group compared with the DCB group in infrapopliteal lesions. Despite the higher restenosis in the DCB group, there was no statistically significant difference in functional outcomes between the two groups.[28] Steiner and colleagues[29] specifically examined the Lutonix DCB device for symptomatic infrapopliteal lesions and found that it was a safe and effective device to use for infrapopliteal lesions, with less than 1% procedural complications and an improvement in Rutherford greater than or equal to 1 category in 59% at 1-year follow-up.

ONGOING TRIALS

Although the superiority of DCBs in treatment of femoropopliteal lesions has been established, the data for infrapopliteal lesions are much less consistent. There are numerous reasons that may explain the discrepancy in outcomes between these two arterial distributions. Lesion complexity tends to be higher in the infrapopliteal distribution, as mentioned previously. Worse distal run-off in this region likely contributes to worse outcomes, and the complexities of postprocedure wound care in CLI seen in many of these patients are a challenge. Another possible explanation is the longer distance the balloon must travel through the bloodstream, shedding paclitaxel before it reaches its destination. Several factors may be involved in the amount of paclitaxel that is deposited at the target site, including the conformation of the uninflated balloon and proximal vessel tortuosity. Additional randomized controlled trials are needed to clarify the role of DCB in this region.

Current studies on DCBs are focused on combination therapies involving the use of DCBs with other treatment modalities (atherectomy and stents) (Table 2). Plaque debulking may allow improved delivery of paclitaxel to the target site. The ADCAT (Atherectomy and Drug-Coated Balloon Angioplasty in Treatment of Long Infrapopliteal Lesions NCT01763476) study is randomizing patients with long (≥60 mm) denovo infrapopliteal lesions to DCB or atherectomy plus DCB, with follow-up angiography at 3 months to assess the rate of binary restenosis. The DEFINITIVE AR (Atherectomy Followed by a Drug Coated Balloon to Treat Peripheral Arterial Disease; NCT01366482) study is evaluating the role of atherectomy before DCB in above and below the knee lesions compared with DCB alone during an extended 2-year follow-up period. One-year data showed lower restenosis in the atherectomy + DCB group compared with DCB alone, although the trial was underpowered for this end point.[30] A third trial, the ISAR-STATH (Efficacy Study of Stenting, Paclitaxel Eluting Balloon or Atherectomy to Treat Peripheral Artery Disease; NCT00986752), is comparing three treatment strategies for PAD: (1) BMS, (2) DCB + BMS, and (3) atherectomy. Six-month results demonstrated lower diameter stenosis in the DCB + BMS compared with stent alone (34.1% vs 55.6%; $P<.01$).[31] The long-term results of these trials will help define the role of plaque debulking before antiproliferative treatment with DCBs.

As shown in the DEBATE-SFA trial,[15] the benefits of stenting and DCB can be combined. Several ongoing studies are comparing DCB + BMS with BMS alone, such as the RAPID (RAndomized Trial of Legflow Paclltaxel Eluting Balloon with Stent Placement versus StanDard Percutaneous Transluminal Angioplasty with Stent Placement for the Treatment of Intermediate [>5 cm and <15 cm] and long [>15 cm] Lesions of the Superficial Femoral Artery; ISRCTN47846578) and the BAIR (Paclitaxel-Coated versus Uncoated Balloon for Treatment of Below-the-Knee In-Stent Restenosis; NCT01398033). However, randomized studies directly comparing DCB with BMS are lacking.

FUTURE DIRECTIONS

Although outcomes with DCB in the femoropopliteal region are promising, the ideal treatment strategy for lesions in the infrapopliteal arterial distribution remains an unmet need. In addition, the ideal antiplatelet regimen after peripheral arterial interventions, including DCB, has not been adequately defined. This question is being addressed by the on-going randomized ASPIRE (Antiplatelet Strategy for Peripheral Arterial Interventions for Revascularization of Lower Extremities; NCT02217501) trial, which will compare outcomes with 1 month versus 12 months of dual-antiplatelet drug treatment. Particular emphasis in this trial is on clinical end points, particularly freedom from repeat revascularization, amputation, and major adverse cardiovascular events.

Future iterations of the DCB will likely include improved drug formulations, allowing for greater efficacy and limiting systemic toxic effects.

Table 2
Ongoing trials of paclitaxel-coated balloons

Trial Name	Total N	DCB Model, n	Formulation, Dose	Control, n	1° Endpoint
Above the knee					
FREERIDE	280	Freeway	Paclitaxel-shellac, 3.0	PTA	6 mo TLR
Advance 18PTX	150	Advance 18PTX	Paclitaxel, 3.0	PTA	6 mo LLL
ISAR-STATH	150	Paclitaxel	Paclitaxel, N/A	PTA + BMS or atherectomy	6 mo % stenosis
COPA CABANA	112	Cotavance	Paclitaxel-iopromide, 3.0	PTA	6 mo LLL
RAPID	176	Legflow	Paclitaxel-shellac + BMS, 3.0	PTA + BMS	24 mo BRS
Definitive AR[a]	53	Cotavance	Paclitaxel-iopromide, 3.0	Atherectomy + Cotavance, paclitaxel-urea, 3.0	12 mo PP; 24 mo MAE
REAL PTX	150	Paclitaxel	N/A	Zilver PTX DCS	12 mo PP
Below the knee					
LUTONIX-BTK	480	Lutonix DCB Moxy	Paclitaxel-polysorbate/sorbitol, 2.0	PTA	12 mo LS; 12 mo PP; freedom from BTK MALE + POD
ADCAT	80	IN.PACT	Paclitaxel-urea, 3.0	Atherectomy + IN.PACT, paclitaxel-urea, 3.0	6 mo PP
RANGER-BTK	30	Ranger SL	Paclitaxel, N/A	N/A	6 mo PP

Abbreviations: BRS, binary restenosis; BTK MALE, below the knee major adverse limb event; DCS, drug-coated stent; LS, limb salvage; MAE, major adverse event rate; POD, postoperative death within 30 days; PP, primary patency.
[a] Two-year follow-up extension study.

The importance of specific excipients is being explored. Furthermore, there is potential for improved cost-effectiveness with the use of DCB.[32] A large meta-analysis showed that compared with PTA, use of DCB was associated with reduction of restenosis from 36.2% to 17.6%, represented greater reduction than with BMS or DES, at a lower incremental cost compared with BMS or DES.[33] Cost-based analyses of treatment strategies explore an increasingly important aspect of medical care, and will no doubt factor into the future of DCBs.

REFERENCES

1. Tendera M, Aboyans V, Bartelink ML, et al. ESC Guidelines on the diagnosis and treatment of peripheral artery diseases. Document covering atherosclerotic disease of extracranial carotid and vertebral, mesenteric, renal, upper and lower extremity arteries: the Task Force on the Diagnosis and Treatment of Peripheral Artery Diseases of the European Society of Cardiology (ESC). Eur Heart J 2011;32:2851–906.

2. Laird JR, Schneider PA, Tepe G, et al. Durability of treatment effect using a drug-coated balloon for femoropopliteal lesions: 24-month results of IN.PACT SFA. J Am Coll Cardiol 2015;66:2329–38.

3. Scheinert D, Scheinert S, Sax J, et al. Prevalence and clinical impact of stent fractures after femoropopliteal stenting. J Am Coll Cardiol 2005;45: 312–5.

4. Rocha-Singh KJ, Jaff MR, Crabtree TR, et al. Performance goals and endpoint assessments for

clinical trials of femoropopliteal bare nitinol stents in patients with symptomatic peripheral arterial disease. Catheter Cardiovasc Interv 2007; 69:910–9.

5. Duda SH, Bosiers M, Lammer J, et al. Drug-eluting and bare nitinol stents for the treatment of atherosclerotic lesions in the superficial femoral artery: long-term results from the SIROCCO trial. J Endovasc Ther 2006;13:701–10.

6. Dake MD, Ansel GM, Jaff MR, et al. Sustained safety and effectiveness of paclitaxel-eluting stents for femoropopliteal lesions: 2-year follow-up from the Zilver PTX randomized and single-arm clinical studies. J Am Coll Cardiol 2013;61: 2417–27.

7. Scheller B, Speck U, Schmitt A, et al. Addition of paclitaxel to contrast media prevents restenosis after coronary stent implantation. J Am Coll Cardiol 2003;42:1415–20.

8. Speck U, Scheller B, Abramjuk C, et al. Neointima inhibition: comparison of effectiveness of non-stent-based local drug delivery and a drug-eluting stent in porcine coronary arteries. Radiology 2006;240: 411–8.

9. Tepe G, Zeller T, Albrecht T, et al. Local delivery of paclitaxel to inhibit restenosis during angioplasty of the leg. N Engl J Med 2008;358:689–99.

10. Werk M, Langner S, Reinkensmeier B, et al. Inhibition of restenosis in femoropopliteal arteries: paclitaxel-coated versus uncoated balloon: femoral paclitaxel randomized pilot trial. Circulation 2008; 118:1358–65.

11. Scheinert D, Duda S, Zeller T, et al. The LEVANT I (Lutonix paclitaxel-coated balloon for the prevention of femoropopliteal restenosis) trial for femoropopliteal revascularization: first-in-human randomized trial of low-dose drug-coated balloon versus uncoated balloon angioplasty. JACC Cardiovasc Interv 2014;7:10–9.

12. Werk M, Albrecht T, Meyer DR, et al. Paclitaxel-coated balloons reduce restenosis after femoropopliteal angioplasty: evidence from the randomized PACIFIER trial. Circ Cardiovasc Interv 2012;5:831–40.

13. Mauri L, Orav EJ, Candia SC, et al. Robustness of late lumen loss in discriminating drug-eluting stents across variable observational and randomized trials. Circulation 2005;112:2833–9.

14. Micari A, Cioppa A, Vadala G, et al. 2-year results of paclitaxel-eluting balloons for femoropopliteal artery disease: evidence from a multicenter registry. JACC Cardiovasc Interv 2013;6:282–9.

15. Liistro F, Grotti S, Porto I, et al. Drug-eluting balloon in peripheral intervention for the superficial femoral artery: the DEBATE-SFA randomized trial (drug eluting balloon in peripheral intervention for the superficial femoral artery). JACC Cardiovasc Interv 2013;6:1295–302.

16. Rosenfield K, Jaff MR, White CJ, et al. Trial of a paclitaxel-coated balloon for femoropopliteal artery disease. N Engl J Med 2015;373:145–53.

17. McKeown LA. Longer term, IN.PACT SFA trial and global registry continue to support DCB Therapy as an option. Conference News VIVA 2016. Available at: https://www.tctmd.com/news/longer-term-inpact-sfa-trial-and-global-registry-continue-support-dcb-therapy-option. Accessed September 26, 2016.

18. Krankenberg H, Tubler T, Ingwersen M, et al. Drug-coated balloon versus standard balloon for superficial femoral artery in-stent restenosis: the randomized femoral artery in-stent restenosis (FAIR) trial. Circulation 2015;132:2230–6.

19. Scheinert D, Schulte KL, Zeller T, et al. Paclitaxel-releasing balloon in femoropopliteal lesions using a BTHC excipient: twelve-month results from the BIOLUX P-I randomized trial. J Endovasc Ther 2015;22:14–21.

20. Schroeder H, Meyer DR, Lux B, et al. Two-year results of a low-dose drug-coated balloon for revascularization of the femoropopliteal artery: outcomes from the ILLUMENATE first-in-human study. Catheter Cardiovasc Interv 2015;86: 278–86.

21. Micari A, Vadala G, Castriota F, et al. 1-year results of paclitaxel-coated balloons for long femoropopliteal artery disease: evidence from the SFA-long study. JACC Cardiovasc Interv 2016;9:950–6.

22. Lyden SP. Built on results: stellarex DCB outcomes from the ILLUMENATE clinical program: insights from ILLUMNATE FIH Study 2-year Results. Paper Presented at: Transcatheter Cardiovascular Therapeutics (TCT). Washington, DC, November 01, 2016.

23. Tepe G, Laird J, Schneider P, et al. Drug-coated balloon versus standard percutaneous transluminal angioplasty for the treatment of superficial femoral and popliteal peripheral artery disease: 12-month results from the IN.PACT SFA randomized trial. Circulation 2015;131:495–502.

24. Schmidt A, Piorkowski M, Werner M, et al. First experience with drug-eluting balloons in infrapopliteal arteries: restenosis rate and clinical outcome. J Am Coll Cardiol 2011;58:1105–9.

25. Liistro F, Porto I, Angioli P, et al. Drug-eluting balloon in peripheral intervention for below the knee angioplasty evaluation (DEBATE-BTK): a randomized trial in diabetic patients with critical limb ischemia. Circulation 2013;128:615–21.

26. Zeller T, Baumgartner I, Scheinert D, et al. Drug-eluting balloon versus standard balloon angioplasty for infrapopliteal arterial revascularization in critical limb ischemia: 12-month results from the IN.PACT DEEP randomized trial. J Am Coll Cardiol 2014;64:1568–76.

27. Zeller T, Beschorner U, Pilger E, et al. Paclitaxel-coated balloon in infrapopliteal arteries: 12-month results from the BIOLUX P-II Randomized Trial (BIOTRONIK'S-First in Man study of the Passeo-18 LUX drug releasing PTA Balloon Catheter vs. the uncoated Passeo-18 PTA balloon catheter in subjects requiring revascularization of infrapopliteal arteries). JACC Cardiovasc Interv 2015;8:1614–22.

28. Siablis D, Kitrou PM, Spiliopoulos S, et al. Paclitaxel-coated balloon angioplasty versus drug-eluting stenting for the treatment of infrapopliteal long-segment arterial occlusive disease: the IDEAS randomized controlled trial. JACC Cardiovasc Interv 2014;7:1048–56.

29. Steiner S, Schmidt A, Bausback Y, et al. Single-center experience with lutonix drug-coated balloons in infrapopliteal arteries. J Endovasc Ther 2016;23: 417–23.

30. Zeller T. DEFINITIVE AR, a multinational pilot study evaluating the effectiveness of directional atherectomy and antirestenotic therapy. Paper Presented at: VIVA. Las Vegas (NV), November 4, 2014.

31. Fusaro M, on behalf of the ISAR-STATH Investigators. Intravascular stenting and angiographic results: randomized comparison of STenting, Stenting after Paclitaxel-eluting balloon and ATHerectomy in patients with symptomatic peripheral artery disease -results at 6 months. Paper Presented at: Leipzig Interventional Course. Leipzig, January 24, 2015.

32. Jeon-Slaughter H, Mohammad A, Haagan D, et al. Direct procedure cost and 30-day outcomes of drug-coated balloon use in femoropopliteal intervention: insights from the XLPAD registry. Chicago: American College of Cardiology; 2016.

33. Katsanos K, Geisler BP, Garner AM, et al. Economic analysis of endovascular drug-eluting treatments for femoropopliteal artery disease in the UK. BMJ Open 2016;6:e011245.

Nitinol Self-Expanding Stents for the Superficial Femoral Artery

Ashwin Nathan, MD[a,b,1], Taisei Kobayashi, MD[a,b,1],
Jay Giri, MD, MPH[a,b,*]

KEYWORDS

- Nitinol • Self-expanding stents • Superficial femoral artery • Peripheral arterial disease

KEY POINTS

- Atherosclerotic vascular disease in the superficial femoral artery is difficult to treat given the biomechanical loading environment of the artery as it courses through the leg.
- Nitinol has material properties that allow it be uniquely suited to withstanding the stresses of stents placed in the superficial femoral artery.
- Novel iterations of self-expanding stents using nitinol have targeted reductions in restenosis and stent fracture.

INTRODUCTION

The superficial femoral artery (SFA) poses unique challenges for endovascular stenting. It is a long, muscular artery that is fixed between the hip and the knee; as a result of the complex motions of the hip joint, the SFA is subject to unique forces, including flexion, extension, and torsion (Fig. 1). The SFA is further exposed to longitudinal and lateral compressional forces and even extrinsic muscular compression as the artery dives through the Hunter canal between the muscular bodies of the anterior and medial compartments of the thigh.[1] Because of the magnitude of mechanical stressors that it is exposed to, the SFA has a particularly prominent smooth muscle layer that allows it to withstand these forces.

Angioplasty alone for atherosclerotic SFA disease is unsuccessful in 30% or more of cases because of the elastic recoil, vascular dissection, and high-grade residual stenosis (Fig. 2).[1]

Balloon-expandable stents were designed to improve patency after SFA angioplasty through the deployment of a metallic lattice that could resist extrinsic forces; although they did decrease failure rates immediately after the procedure, early iterations of these stents were plagued by restenosis and crush damage over time.[2–4]

As a result, alloys were developed that could withstand the stresses of the SFA and were incorporated into self-expanding stents that constantly applied an outward radial force. Early self-expanding stents used Elgiloy, an alloy consisting mainly of cobalt, chromium, and nickel. Initial experiences with self-expanding Elgiloy stents were marked by excessively high rates of stent fracture and low long-term patency. The introduction of a novel material, nitinol, revolutionized treatment of the SFA via improvement in radial strength and incorporation of shape-memory characteristics that promoted crush recovery.[5,6]

Disclosure Statement: The authors have nothing to disclose.
[a] Cardiovascular Medicine Division, Perelman Center, Hospital of the University of Pennsylvania, South Tower, 11th Floor, 3400 Civic Center Boulevard, Philadelphia, PA 19104, USA; [b] Penn Cardiovascular Quality, Outcomes, and Evaluative Research Center, University of Pennsylvania, Philadelphia, PA, USA
[1] These authors are equally contributed.
* Corresponding author. Cardiovascular Medicine Division, Perelman Center, Hospital of the University of Pennsylvania, South Tower, 11th Floor, 3400 Civic Center Boulevard, Philadelphia, PA 19104.
E-mail address: Jay.Giri@uphs.upenn.edu

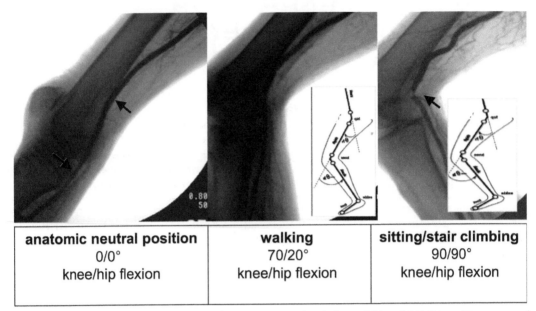

anatomic neutral position 0/0° knee/hip flexion	walking 70/20° knee/hip flexion	sitting/stair climbing 90/90° knee/hip flexion

Fig. 1. Biomechanical loading conditions that the SFA is exposed to during activities of daily living with corresponding angiograms. Blue arrows identify areas of the distal SFA and popliteal artery that are vulnerable to flexion stress.

TECHNICAL CHARACTERISTICS OF NITINOL STENTS

Conventional metal alloys, such as stainless steel or cobalt alloys, provide poor elasticity (1% deformation capability) in comparison with nitinol, which can tolerate 10% strain forces and still retain its original shape.[7] Most elasticity of other metals is reliant on stretching of atomic bonds, but deformational changes to nitinol result in alteration of its crystalline structure. This crystal structure reverts back to its normal shape after the stresses are released. Another key trait of nitinol is that it is temperature sensitive. At low temperatures the frame is easily manipulated, but at body temperature the frame will expand to its original shape and size. This property allows the nitinol stent to be crimped at room temperature and to revert back to its cylindrical shape when deployed in the body.

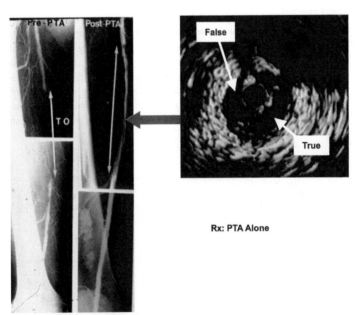

Fig. 2. Intravascular ultrasound of SFA after balloon angioplasty alone. The true lumen and false lumen are clearly seen with intravascular imaging. The arrow identifies the angiographic area shown in the IVUS image. PTA, percutaneous transluminal angioplasty; Rx, prescription.

The manufacturers for nitinol stents can set the temperatures at which the stent becomes more rigid; thus, different stents can exhibit different radial strengths. In other words, some manufacturers may choose to favor more flexibility to avoid stent fracture but will sacrifice some radial strength in doing so.[7,8] Data comparing the differences in radial strengths of commonly used commercially available stents are not readily available.

Original nitinol stents were wire- or sheet-based designs that were welded together to form a tube, but most contemporary nitinol stents are now made from a single tube that is laser cut to create different cell sizes and shapes to create a matrix of metal. As these data regarding cell sizes and shapes are also not currently readily available, it is unclear if these differences in design or cell sizes have an impact on outcomes in the SFA. Comparative effectiveness research of stents with varying technical characteristics has been performed for stents used in the carotid circulation, but further research is warranted in the SFA.[9–11]

EVIDENCE SUPPORTING NITINOL SELF-EXPANDING STENTS

Several major clinical trials demonstrated the benefit of self-expanding nitinol stent (SES) implantation over angioplasty alone for stenosis or occlusion of the SFA (Table 1).

Schillinger and colleagues[12] randomized 104 patients with severe claudication or critical limb ischemia due to stenosis or occlusion of SFA to SES (Dynalink or Absolute Stents [Abbott Vascular, Santa Clara, CA]) or angioplasty with optional secondary stenting. Secondary stenting was performed in 32% of patients randomized to angioplasty, consistent with prior rates of immediate angioplasty failure. At 6 months, restenosis occurred in 24% randomized to primary stenting versus 43% in the angioplasty group (P<.05), as determined by angiography. At 12 months, restenosis occurred in 37% of patients in the stent group and in 63% of angioplasty groups (P = .01), as determined by duplex ultrasonography. Similar improvements in patency were seen in trials by Dick and colleagues[13] using (Biotronik, Berlin, Germany) and the RESILIENT (Randomized Study Comparing the Edwards Self-Expanding LifeStent vs. Angioplasty-Alone In LEsions INvolving The SFA and/or Proximal Popliteal Artery) trial by Laird and colleagues[14] using LifeStents (Bard, Tempe, AZ).

The RESILIENT trial showed an 87.0% freedom from target lesion revascularization (TLR) at 12 months with primary stenting, as compared with 45.1% with angioplasty (P<.001).[13] At 3 years, the difference was persistent, with freedom from TLR in 75.5% versus 41.8% in the stenting and angioplasty groups, respectively.[15]

Table 1
Commercially available stents for the superficial femoral artery

Study	Stent	Subjects	Avg Lesion Length (cm)	CTO (%)	Freedom from TLR	Fracture Rate (%)	12-mo Primary Patency
Leipzig	Supera (Abbott Vascular, Abbott Park, IL)	107	10.9	30	—	0	86
Zilver Trial	Zilver PTX (Cook Medical, Bloomington, IN)	489	6.6	—	—	0.9	83
Sirocco II	S.M.A.R.T. (DES) (Cordis Corporation, Hialeah, FL)	57	8.1	—	91	8.0	82
RESILIENT	LifeStent (Bard, Tempe, AZ)	134	6.2	17	83	3.4	80
Durability	EverFlex (Medtronic, Minneapolis, MN)	151	9.6	40	79	8.1	72
FAST	Luminexx (Bard, Tempe, AZ)	244	4.5	37	85	12.0	67
Super-SL	S.M.A.R.T.	96	13.4	—	75	23.0	65
Vienna	Absolute (Abbott Vascular, Santa Clara, CA)	104	13.0	37	54.3	2.0	63
Vibrant	Bare SES arm	76	16.0	50+	—	>30	58

Lesion length, percentage of chronic total occlusions treated in trial, freedom from target lesion revascularization, fracture rate, and 12-month patency are presented.

Abbreviations: Avg, average; CTO, chronic total occlusions; DES, drug-eluting stent; TLR, target lesion revascularization.

Stent fracture was observed in 3.1% of stents implanted at 12 months.

These studies revealed that using SES in the SFA was more effective in both the short- and long-term when compared with isolated balloon angioplasty. Clinical efficacy data gathered from a wide array of pivotal studies of SFA SES are presented in Table 1.

LESION CHARACTERISTICS ASSOCIATED WITH RESTENOSIS

Registry data demonstrate a large variation in restenosis rates, from as little as 2% for Dynalink and Absolute stents to 28% for Cordis S.M.A.R.T. stents (Cordis Corporation, Hialeah, FL).[16–21] Variation in timing and rigor of follow-up account for some of the wide disparity in reported restenosis rates. However, several patient and procedural factors may contribute to and may predict higher rates of restenosis. Historically, most are patient factors: female sex, diabetes, end-stage renal disease on hemodialysis, Trans-Atlantic Inter-Society Consensus Document II C/D lesions, longer lesion length, and the presence of stent fracture.[5,12,13,20,22–28] These patient-related characteristics in addition to some intraprocedural factors, such as the number of patent tibial vessel runoff at the end of the procedure and stent length, may also predict higher rates of restenosis.[29]

Recent advances in intraprocedural imaging and functional testing may help predict restenosis. One such technique is intravascular ultrasound (IVUS); in one study a minimal luminal area (MLA) of less than 15.5 mm^2 at the end of the procedure was correlated with a higher rate of in-stent restenosis.[30] In practice, a smaller MLA may be a surrogate marker for the degree of difficulty of the intervened-on segment. In other words, heavily calcified arteries or lesions that are resistant to prelesion preparation with scoring balloons or atherectomy devices are less likely to expand and, thus, may be more likely to develop restenosis. Another predictor for restenosis is the use of fractional flow reserve (FFR), which measures the pressure difference across the deployed stent at a state of maximal hyperemia to understand the physiologic significance of residual stenosis.[31] In one study, a poststent FFR value of less than 0.92 predicted a 35.7% risk of restenosis at 1 year versus 4.5% in FFR values greater than 0.92. These two methods show promise for optimizing procedural performance. However, large-scale randomized data regarding their use in the SFA are not yet available.

Synthesis of many of these factors may result in a simple risk stratification model recently proposed by Tsuchiya and colleagues.[32] On analysis, predictors for in-stent restenosis of the SFA were diabetes, current hemodialysis treatment, lack of IVUS investigation, intervention on a chronic total occlusion, and the administration of cilostazol. Patients at low risk of restenosis had 0 to 2 factors present with high-risk patients exhibiting 4 to 5 factors. In this review, low risk patients had a primary patency rate of 66.0% versus 26.3% in high-risk patients. Future risk-modeling work could incorporate additional factors thought to influence restenosis including stent length, utilization of overlapping stents, and the presence of heavy calcification.

STENT FRACTURE

Stent fractures remain a concern, as data suggest that severe fractures may lead to significant restenosis or stent occlusion (Fig. 3).[20,27,33] A seminal article by Scheinert and colleagues[27] revealed that 30% of stent fractures lead to in-stent restenosis and 30% result in total occlusions. In this investigation, longer lesions and utilization of multiple stents were associated with greater risk of stent fracture. When primary patency rates at 1 year were compared between

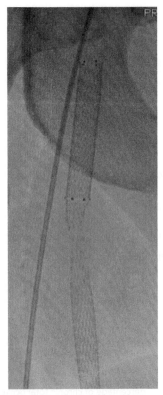

Fig. 3. Fluoroscopic image of complete transverse stent fracture with discontinuity of stent apparent.

fractured and nonfractured stents, nonfractured stents had 84.3% primary patency versus 41.4% in fractured stents.

DEVELOPMENT OF DRUG-ELUTING SELF-EXPANDING NITINOL STENTS

The success of drug-eluting stents (DES) in coronary artery disease led to the adaptation of this technology for SES in the SFA.

Most recently, 5-year data on the largest randomized trial regarding self-expanding DES, Zilver PTX (Cook Medical, Bloomington, IN), versus standard care were published.[34] The Zilver PTX DES is an SES that has a coating of paclitaxel along its outer surfaces. The trial had a unique protocol. Patients were randomized to Zilver PTX versus isolated angioplasty. If patients had an acute failed angioplasty (defined as a >30% residual stenosis or 5 mm Hg mean translesion gradient), secondary randomization was performed to bare SES versus Zilver PTX. The best measure to isolate the effect of the paclitaxel coating involved examination of this secondary randomization group that comprised 120 total patients. Five-year target lesion revascularization rates were numerically lower in the Zilver PTX group, narrowly missing statistical significance (15.1% vs 28.4%, $P = .06$). The study led to Food and Drug Administration (FDA) approval of the Zilver PTX for treatment of de novo SFA disease and has spurred innovation in this area through the industry at large.

STATE-OF-THE-ART DESIGN OF SELF-EXPANDING NITINOL FRAMES

The SFA poses several challenges if the diseased portion of the vessel involves areas of particularly high flexion (distal SFA or involvement of common femoral artery/popliteal artery) with these areas at increased risk of stent fracture, which affect primary patency rates (Fig. 4). The Supera stent

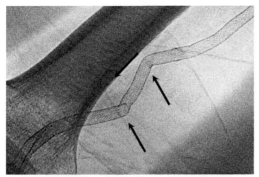

Cross-table lateral knee flexed

Fig. 4. Buckling of distal SFA stent (*arrows*) seen with knee flexion on fluoroscopy.

(Abbott Vascular, Abbott Park, IL) has a unique design that aims to overcome issues related to areas of high flexion. The Supera stent uses 6 pairs of interwoven nitinol wires that are arranged into a helical pattern to create a long tubular stent and stands out from its predecessors for this design change. This stent provides a high degree of flexibility but also superior radial strength compared with its tubular stent competitors.[35]

True comparative effectiveness data with the Supera stent are sparse. However, in the SUPERB (Comparison of the SUpera® PERipheral System in the Superficial Femoral Artery) study primary patency rates at 1 year were 78.9%, with 0% stent fracture in a relatively complex set of lesions.[35] A recent, single-center report of 305 Supera stents placed in 147 patients showed no stent fractures in the popliteal and tibial-peroneal segments in those patients whereby these stents extended into these areas, lending credence to the potential of Supera in this high-flexion area.

The BioMimics 3D stent (Veryan Medical, Oxford, United Kingdom) is an SES that simulates the normal helical nature of arterial anatomy to recreate swirling blood flow in the stented artery. The goal of the stent design is to maintain dynamic shear stress on the arterial wall, a characteristic that has been shown in porcine vessels to decrease intimal hyperplasia and the risk of in-stent restenosis.[36] Zeller and colleagues[36] studied the outcomes of a helical versus a tubular design of SES and showed improved primary patency of the helical over tubular stents at 1 and 2 years (80% vs 71% at 1 year and 72% vs 55% at 2 years). There were corresponding improvements in ankle-brachial indices and Rutherford categories favoring helical-shaped stents.

Recently, the Tigris (W. L. Gore and Associates, Newark, DE) vascular stent was approved by the FDA for the treatment of stenosis in the SFA and proximal popliteal artery. It is a third-generation, dual-component stent that consists of a nitinol stent with an external fluoropolymer lattice that provides flexible and biocompatible interconnections. It has been specifically designed to tolerate the mechanical forces that have previously caused stent fractures at the knee, including extension, compression, flexion, and torsion. Further, it is coated with heparin to prevent thrombus formation. As larger clinical trials using this stent become available, its advantages in reducing stent fracture will be more fully evaluated.

SUMMARY

The SFA is a complex artery with several unique anatomic characteristics that affect stent patency. The characteristics of the nitinol alloy have helped to bridge the gap between flexibility and strength to provide enough support to withstand recoil but to also deliver enough elasticity to flex along with patient movement. These advances have improved the primary patency rates after balloon angioplasty and have quickly become the standard of care for SFA interventions. Novel iterations of the nitinol stent, including drug-eluting versions, and interwoven and helical stent designs show promise for further improving the outcomes in this challenging anatomic area.

REFERENCES

1. Schillinger M, Minar E. Past, present and future of femoropopliteal stenting. J Endovasc Ther 2009; 16(Suppl 1):I147–52.
2. Becquemin JP, Favre JP, Marzelle J, et al. Systematic versus selective stent placement after superficial femoral artery balloon angioplasty: a multicenter prospective randomized study. J Vasc Surg 2003; 37(3):487–94.
3. Grimm J, Müller-Hülsbeck S, Jahnke T, et al. Randomized study to compare PTA alone versus PTA with Palmaz stent placement for femoropopliteal lesions. J Vasc Interv Radiol 2001;12(8):935–42.
4. Cejna M, Thurnher S, Illiasch H, et al. PTA versus Palmaz stent placement in femoropopliteal artery obstructions: a multicenter prospective randomized study. J Vasc Interv Radiol 2001;12(1):23–31.
5. Sabeti S, Mlekusch W, Amighi J, et al. Primary patency of long-segment self-expanding nitinol stents in the femoropopliteal arteries. J Endovasc Ther 2005;12(1):6–12.
6. Sabeti S, Schillinger M, Amighi J, et al. Primary patency of femoropopliteal arteries treated with nitinol versus stainless steel self-expanding stents: propensity score-adjusted analysis. Radiology 2004;232(2):516–21.
7. Stoeckel D, Pelton A, Duerig T. Self-expanding nitinol stents: material and design considerations. Eur Radiol 2004;14(2):292–301.
8. Duda SH, Wiskirchen J, Tepe G, et al. Physical properties of endovascular stents: an experimental comparison. J Vasc Interv Radiol 2000;11(5):645–54.
9. Stabile E, Giugliano G, Cremonesi A, et al. Impact on outcome of different types of carotid stent: results from the European Registry of Carotid Artery Stenting. EuroIntervention 2016;12(2):e265–70.
10. Park KY, Kim DI, Kim BM, et al. Incidence of embolism associated with carotid artery stenting: open-cell versus closed-cell stents. J Neurosurg 2013; 119(3):642–7.
11. Doig D, Turner EL, Dobson J, et al. Predictors of stroke, myocardial infarction or death within 30 days of carotid artery stenting: results from the International Carotid Stenting Study. Eur J Vasc Endovasc Surg 2016;51(3):327–34.
12. Schillinger M, Sabeti S, Loewe C, et al. Balloon angioplasty versus implantation of nitinol stents in the superficial femoral artery. N Engl J Med 2006; 354(18):1879–88.
13. Laird JR, Katzen BT, Scheinert D, et al. Nitinol stent implantation versus balloon angioplasty for lesions in the superficial femoral artery and proximal popliteal artery: twelve-month results from the RESILIENT randomized trial. Circ Cardiovasc Interv 2010;3(3):267–76.
14. Dick P, Wallner H, Sabeti S, et al. Balloon angioplasty versus stenting with nitinol stents in intermediate length superficial femoral artery lesions. Catheter Cardiovasc Interv 2009;74(7):1090–5.
15. Laird JR, Katzen BT, Scheinert D, et al. Nitinol stent implantation vs. balloon angioplasty for lesions in the superficial femoral and proximal popliteal arteries of patients with claudication: three-year follow-up from the RESILIENT randomized trial. J Endovasc Ther 2012;19(1):1–9.
16. Sakamoto Y, Hirano K, Iida O, et al. Five-year outcomes of self-expanding nitinol stent implantation for chronic total occlusion of the superficial femoral and proximal popliteal artery. Catheter Cardiovasc Interv 2013;82(3):E251–6.
17. Laird JR, Jain A, Zeller T, et al. Nitinol stent implantation in the superficial femoral artery and proximal popliteal artery: twelve-month results from the complete SE multicenter trial. J Endovasc Ther 2014;21(2):202–12.
18. Nasser F, Kambara A, Abath C, et al. Safety and efficacy of the EPIC™ Nitinol Vascular Stent System for the treatment of lesions located in the superficial femoral artery: prospective and multicentric trial. J Cardiovasc Surg (Torino) 2015. [Epub ahead of print].
19. Lichtenberg M, Kolks O, Hailer B, et al. PEACE I all-comers registry: patency evaluation after implantation of the 4-French Pulsar-18 self-expanding nitinol stent in femoropopliteal lesions. J Endovasc Ther 2014;21(3):373–80.
20. Lin Y, Tang X, Fu W, et al. Stent fractures after superficial femoral artery stenting: risk factors and impact on patency. J Endovasc Ther 2015;22(3): 319–26.
21. Vardi M, Novack V, Pencina MJ, et al. Safety and efficacy metrics for primary nitinol stenting in femoropopliteal occlusive disease: a meta-analysis and critical examination of current methodologies. Catheter Cardiovasc Interv 2014;83(6):975–83.
22. Iida O, Uematsu M, Soga Y, et al. Timing of the restenosis following nitinol stenting in the superficial femoral artery and the factors associated with early and late restenoses. Catheter Cardiovasc Interv 2011;78(4):611–7.

23. Razzouk L, Aggarwal S, Gorgani F, et al. In-stent restenosis in the superficial femoral artery. Ann Vasc Surg 2013;27(4):510–24.

24. Cheng SW, Ting AC, Wong J. Endovascular stenting of superficial femoral artery stenosis and occlusions: results and risk factor analysis. Cardiovasc Surg 2001;9(2):133–40.

25. Rocha-Singh KJ, Jaff MR, Crabtree TR, et al, VIVA Physicians Inc. Performance goals and endpoint assessments for clinical trials of femoropopliteal bare nitinol stents in patients with symptomatic peripheral arterial disease. Catheter Cardiovasc Interv 2007; 69(6):910–9.

26. Duda SH, Pusich B, Richter G, et al. Sirolimus-eluting stents for the treatment of obstructive superficial femoral artery disease: six-month results. J Invasive Cardiol 2004;16(Suppl A):15A–9A.

27. Scheinert D, Scheinert S, Sax J, et al. Prevalence and clinical impact of stent fractures after femoropopliteal stenting. J Am Coll Cardiol 2005;45(2):312–5.

28. Bakken AM, Palchik E, Hart JP, et al. Impact of diabetes mellitus on outcomes of superficial femoral artery endoluminal interventions. J Vasc Surg 2007;46(5):946–58 [discussion: 958].

29. Ihnat DM, Duong ST, Taylor ZC, et al. Contemporary outcomes after superficial femoral artery angioplasty and stenting: the influence of TASC classification and runoff score. J Vasc Surg 2008; 47(5):967–74.

30. Miki K, Fujii K, Kawasaki D, et al. Intravascular ultrasound-derived stent dimensions as predictors of angiographic restenosis following nitinol stent implantation in the superficial femoral artery. J Endovasc Ther 2016;23(3):424–32.

31. Kobayashi N, Hirano K, Yamawaki M, et al. Ability of fractional flow reserve to predict restenosis after superficial femoral artery stenting. J Endovasc Ther 2016;23(6):896–902.

32. Tsuchiya T, Takamura T, Soga Y, et al. Clinical impact and risk stratification of balloon angioplasty for femoropopliteal disease in nitinol stenting era: retrospective multicenter study using propensity score matching analysis. SAGE Open Med 2016;4. 2050312116660116.

33. Schlager O, Dick P, Sabeti S, et al. Long-segment SFA stenting–the dark sides: in-stent restenosis, clinical deterioration, and stent fractures. J Endovasc Ther 2005;12(6):676–84.

34. Dake MD, Ansel GM, Jaff MR, et al. Durable clinical effectiveness with paclitaxel-eluting stents in the femoropopliteal artery: 5-year results of the Zilver PTX randomized trial. Circulation 2016;133(15): 1472–83 [discussion: 1483].

35. Garcia L, Jaff MR, Metzger C, et al. Wire-interwoven nitinol stent outcome in the superficial femoral and proximal popliteal arteries: twelve-month results of the SUPERB trial. Circ Cardiovasc Interv 2015;8(5).

36. Zeller T, Gaines PA, Ansel GM, et al. Helical centerline stent improves patency: two-year results from the randomized mimics trial. Circ Cardiovasc Interv 2016;9(6).

Current Role of Atherectomy for Treatment of Femoropopliteal and Infrapopliteal Disease

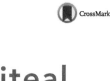

Nicolas W. Shammas, MD, EJD, MS, FSCAI, FICA, FSVM[a,b,c,*]

KEYWORDS

• Atherectomy • Restenosis • Revascularization • Femoropopliteal artery • Infrapopliteal artery
• Distal embolization

KEY POINTS

• Atherectomy improves the acute procedural success of a procedure whether treating de novo or restenotic (including in-stent) disease.
• Intermediate follow-up results seem to be in favor of atherectomy in delaying and reducing the need for repeat revascularization in patients with femoropopliteal in-stent restenosis.
• Recent data suggest that avoiding cutting into the external elastic lamina is an important factor in reducing restenosis.
• The interplay between directional atherectomy and drug-coated balloons is unclear.

INTRODUCTION

Endovascular interventions continue to replace surgery as a first-line therapy for femoropopliteal (FP) and infrapopliteal disease.[1] Randomized trials have shown that patency improves with the use of self-expanding stents in the superficial femoral artery, but there are conflicting data as to whether this leads to reduction in target lesion revascularization (TLR) or improved symptoms and quality of life when compared with balloon angioplasty (percutaneous transluminal angioplasty, PTA).[2–6] Although stenting is appealing to many endovascular specialists because it can be performed with relative ease, higher speed, and predictable excellent angiographic results, the long-term outcome remains a problem with a high rate of restenosis and need for repeat TLR. Also, stent fracture continues to be seen, which may have an impact on restenosis and future therapies.[7]

The concept of an optimal approach for infrainguinal interventions using a no-stent strategy has been recently propelled with the advent of drug-coated balloons (DCB). The concept of changing vessel compliance (C) with atherectomy, protecting the distal vascular bed (P) and applying anti-restenotic drugs (R) to the treated segment, has become a main strategy to treat FP and infrapopliteal disease.[8] This "CPR" concept (Fig. 1) has revived interest in atherectomy as a viable tool to reduce dissection and bailout stenting and to accomplish optimal acute angiographic results[7] in preparation for the application of antiproliferative drugs. The randomized DEFINITIVE AR feasibility trial[9] points to the viability of this concept, which awaits further proof from larger registries and well-powered randomized trials.

Data on DCB have shown superior results to PTA in treating FP disease particularly in short- and intermediate-length lesions.[10–15] Severe calcification was excluded for the most part in these

[a] Midwest Cardiovascular Research Foundation, 1622 E Lombard Street, Davenport, IA 52803, USA; [b] University of Iowa, 200 Hawkins Dr, Iowa City, IA 52242, USA; [c] Genesis Heart Institute, Cardiovascular Medicine, PC, 1236 East Rusholme street, Suite 300, Davenport, IA 52803, USA
* Midwest Cardiovascular Research Foundation, 1622 East Lombard Street, Davenport, IA 52803.
E-mail address: Shammas@mchsi.com

Intervent Cardiol Clin 6 (2017) 235–249
http://dx.doi.org/10.1016/j.iccl.2016.12.007
2211-7458/17/© 2016 Elsevier Inc. All rights reserved.

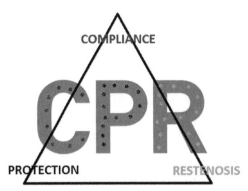

Fig. 1. CPR or the triad of improving Compliance, Protecting the distal vascular bed, and reducing Restenosis as part of an optimal strategy in treating infrainguinal peripheral arterial disease.

studies. In these "simple" lesions, DCB have emerged as a first-line therapy. However, these trials also excluded lesions with high residual narrowing or flow-limiting dissection following pretreatment with PTA. For instance, in the run-in phase of the Levant II trial, 11/56 (19.6%) of patients were excluded.[16] Pretreatment of these lesions, therefore, with atherectomy may improve the chance of avoiding stenting while improving outcome with DCB. The incremental benefit of atherectomy over DCB in these simple lesions, however, needs to be weighed against the added cost of atherectomy.

It is likely that atherectomy's value is in treating complex FP and infrapopliteal disease. There is no uniform classification for complex disease, but operators generally agree that severe calcium, thrombus, long lesions greater than 10 to 15 cm, and total occlusions constitute complex lesions. Both calcium and thrombus are highly prevalent in the FP artery and quite often underdiagnosed angiographically.[17–19] Calcium is likely to be found in atherosclerotic plaques in the FP arteries but also in the media (Monckeberg), particularly in patients with diabetes and chronic renal failure.[17]

Complex disease is quite often a predictor of flow-limiting dissection and stenting.[20] Also, in a small study, Fanelli and colleagues[21] have shown that severe calcium ($\geq 270°$ arc of calcium) reduces the effectiveness of DCB with a higher loss of patency at 1-year follow-up when compared with lesions with mild to moderate calcification. Furthermore, recent data from Tepe and colleagues[22] showed that bilateral calcification in FP disease on angiographic imaging is associated with a higher late lumen loss after DCB. In that study, bilateral calcification at the same lesion level had the most profound impact on late lumen loss instead of the depth of calcium (intimal, medial, or adventitial) or its length. Based on

these findings, bilateral calcium on angiogram at the same lesion level or an arc of calcium of 270° or greater appear to correlate with worse outcomes after DCB. Finally, thrombus has a high affinity to paclitaxel, making it less available to the vessel wall and potentially may reduce its effectiveness.[23]

Atherectomy offers a way to modify complex disease by improving vessel compliance[24–26] and therefore reducing the need for high pressure balloon dilation and barotrauma, leading to a low incidence of flow-limiting dissection and need for stenting. Also, atherectomy may modify the overall milieu of complex plaque by allowing better drug penetration and diffusion into the vessel wall when compared with applying DCB without atherectomy.[27] Furthermore, atherectomy catheters with aspiration capacity (JetStream; Boston Scientific, Maples Grove, MN, USA) or with ablative potential (Excimer laser; Spectranetics, Colorado Springs, CO, USA) have the ability to remove thrombus, which may also have a positive effect on improving drug availability to the vessel wall. Whether these features of atherectomy lead to improvement in clinical outcomes is unclear, and data from future well-powered trials are awaited.

ATHERECTOMY FOR FEMOROPOPLITEAL DE NOVO AND NONSTENT RESTENOTIC DISEASE

Fig. 2 illustrates a proposed algorithm for the treatment of complex de novo and nonstent restenotic disease. This proposed algorithm is based on several registries and small randomized trials as well as the author's experience. Currently, there is no unified consensus on how to approach these lesions among operators.[28] The atherectomy device choice is highly lesion dependent (Fig. 3) but also influenced significantly by device availability and operator experience.

JetStream Atherectomy
The JetStream XC is a rotational cutter with aspiration capacity (Fig. 4). It has significantly been upgraded from its predecessor, the Pathway atherectomy device.[29] The JetStream XC has significantly more cutting and aspiration power and leads to a higher minimal luminal area (MLA) after treatment. The JetStream is suitable for all lesions. However, severely eccentric lesions may be best not treated with this device because of wire bias, particularly in the early experience of the operator. Also, the device is not to be used in iliac, renal, carotid, or coronary arteries as per the instructions for use label. Jet-Stream is effective but off label for treatment

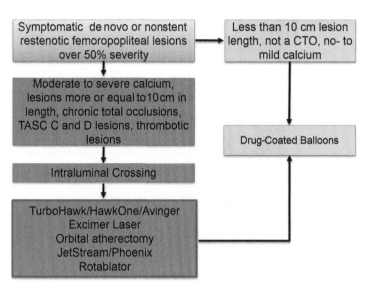

Fig. 2. Proposed algorithm for the management of symptomatic complex de novo or nonstent restenotic FP lesions using atherectomy as a first-line therapy.

of in-stent restenosis (ISR), and this will be addressed in detail in later discussion. JetStream was tested in moderate to severely calcified short lesions (Fig. 5). In the prospective, single-arm JetStream Calcium study,[30] calcium removal was evaluated with intravascular ultrasound (IVUS) pre-JetStream and post-JetStream treatment of FP lesions. In 26 patients that met inclusion criteria, IVUS increased MLA from 6.6 ± 3.7 mm^2 to 10.0 ± 3.6 mm^2 ($P = .001$). Calcium removal accounted for $86\% \pm 23\%$ of the lumen increase after atherectomy. Although no significant distal embolization (DE) was reported in this study, DE can still occur with the JetStream device and ranged from 0% to 9% in different studies. Recently, it has been shown that the use of an embolic filter, particularly the Nav-6 filter (off-label application) (Abbott Vascular

Solutions, Abbott Park, IL, USA), seems to provide, at least numerically, a reduction in significant DE (1.8% vs 8%, $P = .1$).[31] In the JetStream ISR study,[32] no DE occurred with the use of the Nav-6 filter, whereas one-third of DE occurred with the Spider filter (Medtronic, St Paul, MN, USA) and two-thirds with no filters. The author currently uses embolic filter protection (EFP) in patients with severely calcified disease, total occlusions, long lesions greater than 10 cm, thrombotic lesions, and patients with a single infrapopliteal runoff. It should be noted, however, that the use of any filter with the JetStream XC device is currently off label. Finally, the JetStream is also approved as an embolectomy device for thrombus removal. In the author's experience, the JetStream 2.4/3.4 is quite effective in removal of thrombus.

☺ = on label   ☺ = off label   ☻ = Do not use   X = Effective   XX = Very effective

Atherectomy Type	Directional		Rotational		Photo-Ablative		Orbital	
Atherectomy Device	TurboHawk		Jetstream XC		Excimer Laser		Diamondback 360	
Short Eccentric	XX	☺	X	☺	X	☺	X	☺
Thrombus	-	☻	XX	☺	XX	☺	-	☻
Below the knee	X	☺	X	☺	XX	☺	XX	☺
Long calcified disease	X	☺	XX	☺	X	☺	XX	☺
In-stent restenosis	-	☻	XX	☺	XX	☺	-	☻
Chronic total occlusion	XX	☺	XX	☺	XX	☺	XX	☺

Fig. 3. Suggested atherectomy device choices in different lesion subsets.

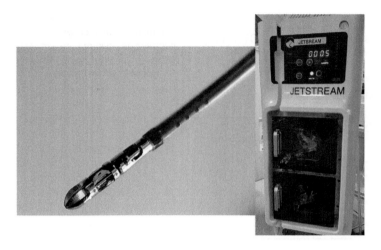

Fig. 4. JetStream XC atherectomy device with Console. (Boston Scientific, Maples Grove, MN.)

Early data on rotational and aspiration atherectomy were published as part of the Pathway PVD trial.[33] In this prospective, single-arm study, 172 patients in Europe were treated with Pathway atherectomy with device success reaching 99% and low bailout stenting of 7%. TLR was reported at 26% at 1 year. The JET registry,[34] a multicenter, prospective, open-label nonrandomized study, has recently completed the 1-year follow-up on 241 patients in 37 US investigational sites. Early data presented in 2015 at CRT from the first 155 patients indicated that the JET registry enrolled real world patients with a mean lesion length of 220 ± 290 mm. The acute procedural success was high at more than 98% (Fig. 6). Post-JetStream and adjunctive PTA residual stenosis was reduced from 99% to 9%. DE requiring treatment was 2% despite only 19% of patients receiving EFP. The full study acute and long-term data (patency and freedom from TLR) will be presented early 2017.

Orbital Atherectomy

Orbital atherectomy (OA; Cardiovascular Systems, Inc, St. Paul, MN, USA) (Fig. 7) uses the eccentric, diamond-coated Diamondback 360° crown mounted on the end of a drive shaft that rotates at different speeds. The higher the speed, the wider the orbit of differential sanding. This device is effective in modifying and sanding calcium but is likely to be less effective in softer plaques and is contraindicated in thrombotic and ISR. Long, diffuse moderate to severe calcified disease can typically be treated with OA with good procedural success and reduced flow limiting dissection and bailout stenting. Applying OA before drug-eluting stents may also lead to better stent expansion and possibly more drug penetration into the vessel wall (Fig. 8). The device typically generates microdebris that is small enough to pass through the capillary system and washes out with no or mild flow

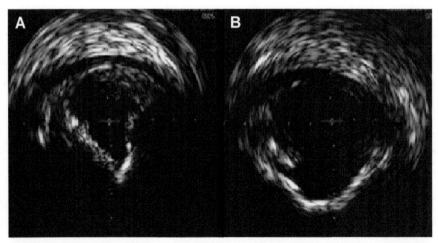

Fig. 5. (A) Pre-JS. (B) Post-JS.

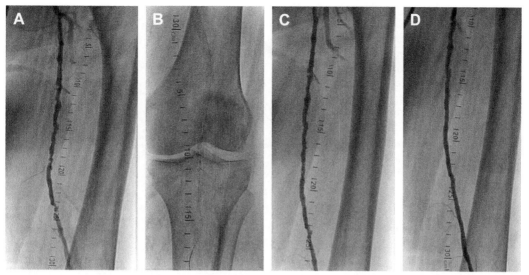

Fig. 6. JS of complex, long irregular disease (A). Filter in place in the P3 segment of the popliteal (B). Post-JetStream only (C). Post-DCB (D).

impairment. EFP are rarely used with OA and generally are not necessary.

In the COMPLIANCE 360° trial,[26] OA reduced dissection (15.8% vs 48.1%, P = .02) and bailout stenting (5.3% vs 77.8%, P<.001) with numerically higher freedom from TLR (81.2% vs 78.3%). Prospective registries also confirmed these acute findings in real-world patients, again confirming a low dissection and stenting rate after plaque modification with OA. In the CONFIRM registry,[35,36] residual narrowing after low pressure adjunctive balloon angioplasty was 10%, and the data were best for severely calcified plaques and least effective for soft plaques. Technique is important to reduce complications as seen in CONFIRM with shorter spin times and use of smaller crown sizes. This technique reduced significantly slow flow (4.4%), embolism (2.2%), and spasm (6.3%). Aggressive debulking is discouraged with OA with the focus primarily on plaque modification to improve vessel compliance and reduce dissection and need for stenting. Finally, data from calcified cadaveric human lower limbs[27] showed that OA-treated segments have an increase in paclitaxel uptake by 20% in the FP vessels and 400% in the tibial arteries with an average increase of drug deposit greater than

50%. Furthermore, paclitaxel extended more diffusely into the treated segments.

The cost-effectiveness of OA in treating FP calcified disease was recently evaluated using data from the COMPLIANCE 360 study. Weinstock and colleagues[37] noted that despite higher hospital charges and costs for OA compared with PTA, there were significant differences in cost for single lesions versus multiple lesions, and the 1-year incremental cost of OA versus PTA alone was US$549 with an incremental quality-adjusted life-year of 0.16. The incremental cost-effectiveness ratio was US$3441 making OA a desirable procedure from a health economic standpoint.

TurboHawk/HawkOne Atherectomy System

In a 2-center, randomized trial of SilverHawk atherectomy (Fig. 9) with adjunctive PTA versus PTA alone in de novo FP disease,[24] directional atherectomy was shown to reduce dissections and bailout stenting by approximately 55%. This study was the first randomized proof-of-concept study that demonstrated the ability of plaque excision to modify vessel compliance and reduce stent need (Fig. 10). The study included 58 patients with 29 vessels (36 vessels) randomized to atherectomy and 29 vessels (48 vessels) randomized to PTA. TLR (16.7% vs 11.1%) and target vessel revascularization (TVR; 21.4% vs 11.1%) were statistically similar between the 2 groups, but bailout stenting was performed in 62.1% in the PTA arm versus 27.6% in the atherectomy arm (P = .017). Distal macroembolization captured by EFP occurred in 11 of 17

Fig. 7. Diamond-coated Diamondback 360° crown mounted eccentrically on the end of the drive shaft. (*Courtesy of* Cardiovascular Systems, Inc, St. Paul, MN.)

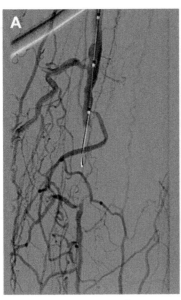
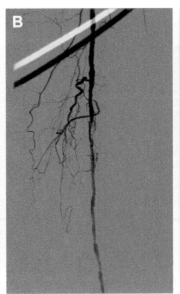
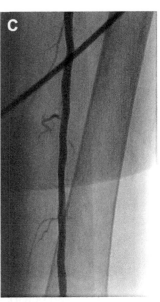

Fig. 8. Crossing superficial femoral artery CTO (*A*). Post-OA alone (*B*). Postangioplasty and stenting with full stent expansion (*C*).

patients (64.7%) treated with atherectomy versus none of 10 in the PTA group (*P*<.001) in patients. The problem of DE with TurboHawk atherectomy was also demonstrated in the Definitive Ca study.[38] In this pivotal multicenter trial of 133 patients (168 subjects) that led to the approval of the SpiderFx Filter when used in conjunction with the TurboHawk in moderately and severely calcified superficial femoral arteries, the filter successfully captured embolic debris in 97.5% (119/122) of cases, but DE requiring additional treatment occurred only in 3 patients. Despite the extent of calcification in the vessels enrolled, the dissection rate was as low as 0.8% (type D and higher) and stenting was required in only 4.1% of cases. This registry also confirmed the

ability of directional atherectomy with the Turbo-Hawk to reduce dissection and bailout stenting confirming the data from the early feasibility study. Furthermore, the multicenter, multinational DEFINITIVE LE (Determination of EFfectiveness of the SilverHawk PerIpheral Plaque ExcisioN System [SIlverHawk Device] for the Treatment of Infrainguinal VEssels/Lower Extremities) registry[39] prospectively enrolled 800 patients. In this registry, lesion length was 8.3 ± 5.5 mm (≥10 cm in 27.8%); chronic total occlusions (CTOs) were 20.8%, and vessel calcification was 37.1%. The 12-month restenosis rate was 22% with no difference between diabetics versus nondiabetics. DE occurred in 3.8%, perforation in 5.3%, and bailout stenting in 3.2%.

Directional atherectomy using the Avinger Optical Coherence Tomography Pantheris system (Fig. 11) provides the ability to cut plaque while avoiding the external elastic lamina (EEL). Recent data indicated that cutting into the EEL increases the rate of restenosis. The VISION IDE trial is a multicenter, nonrandomized study that evaluated the Pantheris system. Early data from VISION[40] showed no dissections or perforations and a stenting rate of 4% with the Pantheris system. Freedom from TLR was 89.2% at 6 months. Long-term and comparative data are still needed, and the device is not optimal for severely calcified disease and may be challenging to use in long lesions.

Data suggest that adjunctive directional atherectomy to DCB may be a promising strategy to

Fig. 9. TurboHawk catheter. (Medtronic, Minneapolis, MN.)

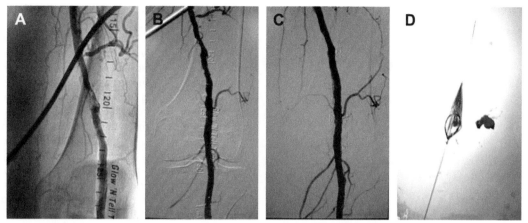

Fig. 10. Eccentric calcified distal superficial femoral artery (*A*). Post-TurboHawk atherectomy with 40% residual narrowing (*B*). Postadjunctive balloon angioplasty with no dissection and less than 10% residual narrowing (*C*). Spider FX Filter with embolic debris captured post-TurboHawk atherectomy (*D*).

improve outcome of endovascular interventions of complex FP arterial disease. In the Definitive AR feasibility study,[9] patients treated with Silver-Hawk atherectomy and DCB (DAART arm) had a tendency toward higher patency in long (>10 cm) and severely calcified disease when compared with DCB alone. This favorable result with DCB after adjunctive SilverHawk atherectomy was also noted in a small observational study (n = 30)[41] that enrolled patients with advanced symptoms (mean Rutherford Becker category of 4.2) and severe calcified peripheral arteries. These patients were treated with IVUS-guided directional atherectomy followed by DCB under embolic protection. In this study, bailout stenting was 6.5% and freedom from TLR was 90%. Finally, the REALITY study (DiRectional AthErectomy + Drug CoAted BaLloon to Treat Long, CalcifIed FemoropopliTeal ArterY Lesions) is currently evaluating the role of SilverHawk atherectomy as an adjunctive treatment to DCB in long, calcified disease (https://clinical-trials.gov/ct2/show/NCT02850107).

Excimer Laser Atherectomy

The xenon chloride excimer laser (pulsed 308-nm system) (**Fig. 12**) is capable of photoablating plaque and thrombus. Its application in complex FP disease is in total chronic occlusions, long lesions, and thrombotic lesions. Also, the laser is approved for ISR, which is discussed later in this article. The excimer laser is not ideal for severe calcified disease.

The laser comes in sizes ranging from 0.9 mm to 2.5 mm with the larger catheters (1.7–2.5 mm) best suited for FP interventions and the smaller

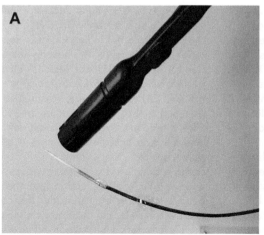

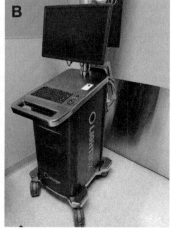

Fig. 11. Pantheris atherectomy system. (*A*) Catheter with handle. (*B*) Console. (Avinger, Redwood City, CA.)

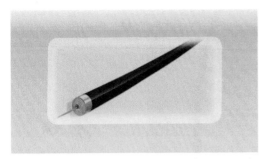

Fig. 12. Excimer laser catheter. (Spectranetics, Colorado Springs, CO.)

ones (0.9–1.4 mm) best suited for infrapopliteal disease, including the pedal arteries. The Turbo Tandem laser can be used as a directional catheter to maximize tissue ablation. Recently, the Turbo-Power laser was also approved for use in de novo and restenotic lesions (including ISR).

Maximum tissue ablation and reduction of DE may be achieved by advancing the catheters slowly at 1 to 2 mm/s. However, DE does occur with excimer laser similar to all atherectomy devices. The Distal Embolic Event Protection Using Excimer Laser Ablation in Peripheral Vascular Interventions (DEEP EMBOLI) study[42] has shown that macroembolization does occur in 66.7% of patients treated with 22.2% exceeding 2 mm in axial length. Also, using continuous Doppler monitoring, Lam and colleagues[43] showed that the average number of embolic signals during FP interventions was 12 for PTA, 28 for stenting, 49 for SilverHawk, and 51 for laser. The size of the debris generating these signals could not be determined. The author continues to use EFP with the laser in complex lesions and patients with single distal runoff.

The multicenter, prospective CliRpath Excimer Laser System to Enlarge Lumen Openings (CELLO) registry[44] enrolled 65 patients with FP arterial disease treated with excimer laser and adjunctive balloon angioplasty or stenting. CTOs was present in 20% of patients, and mean lesion length was 5.6 ± 4.7 cm. TLR at 1 year was 23.1%. This study was not designed to assess change in vessel compliance and rate of stenting after laser treatment. Also, lesions in this study are relatively short and of low complexity.

Scheinert and colleagues[45] reported data on excimer laser in CTOs of the superficial femoral artery. In 318 consecutive patients (411 superficial femoral artery, SFAs), the occlusion length was 19.4 ± 6.0 cm in length. Technical success rate was 90.5% (372/411) with a low rate of acute reocclusion (1.0%), perforation (2.2%),

and DE (3.9%). Bailout stenting was only 7.1%. At 1 year, restenosis however was high at 66.4%. Similarly, the Peripheral Excimer Laser Angioplasty trial[46] was a multicenter, randomized, prospective study of adjunctive laser with PTA versus PTA alone in CTO >10 cm. In this trial, bailout stenting was advised only for flow limiting dissection or significant recoil. Stent utilization was 42% with the laser versus 59% with PTA (P = .02). Also, DE was 3% with the laser versus 9% with PTA alone. At 1 year, patency was similar between the laser and PTA at 49%. The laser, similar to other atherectomy devices, seems to reduce the rate of dissection and bailout stenting in complex disease.

ATHERECTOMY FOR INFRAPOPLITEAL DISEASE

The infrapopliteal arteries have a high prevalence of medial calcification (70% of cases) irrespective of symptoms. The prevalence of severe calcium is higher in men, diabetics, and chronic renal failure and results in bone formation in 10% to 15% of patients.[17,18] Furthermore, calcium in the infrapopliteal vessels can be difficult to dilate and requires high balloon pressure dilation, which may lead to significant dissections and often the need for stenting, best avoided below the knee because of the risk of stent underexpansion, thrombosis, fracture, and lack of data that show reduction in amputations or vascular death. Finally, the severity of calcium below the knee can be a barrier to antiproliferative drug diffusion into the vessel wall.

Orbital Atherectomy

The pivotal OASIS trial[47] was a nonrandomized, prospective multicenter registry that enrolled 124 patients (201 stenoses) with severe infrapopliteal disease. Procedural success (final stenosis less or equal 30%) was 90.1% (see Fig. 14) and the 6-month combined endpoint of death, amputation, or TVR was 10.4%. Despite heavy calcification present in 55% of lesions, stenting was performed only in 2.5% of lesions (Fig. 13). Also, the CALCIUM 360° study,[25] a multicenter, randomized trial of OA with adjunctive PTA versus PTA alone in severely calcified infrapopliteal disease in critical limb ischemia (CLI) patients demonstrated that "differential sanding" of severely calcified vessels improves vessel compliance and reduces dissection rate and the need bailout stenting. In this study, the compliance was evaluated by the maximum balloon pressure required to obtain full balloon inflation after atherectomy (5.9 atm) versus PTA (9.4 atm) (P<.001).

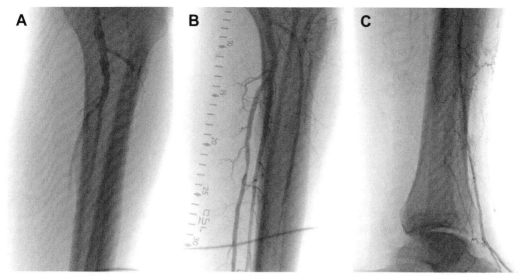

Fig. 13. OA of a total occlusion of the anterior tibialis (A). Post-OA and no adjunctive balloon angioplasty yielding less than 10% residual narrowing (B) with continued good runoff and no DE (C).

Lower barotrauma after OA translated into a higher procedural success rate (93.1% vs 82.4%), less flow-limiting dissections (3.3% vs 11.4%), and need for bailout stenting (6.9% vs 14.3%). Although this study was not powered to evaluate freedom from major adverse events (MAE), patients in the OA arm experienced lower MAE than those in the PTA arm (93.3% vs 57.9%, $P = .006$). This finding was consistent with a recent meta-analysis that showed that atherectomy in conjunction with PTA with or without stenting reduces amputation rates, mortality, and post-procedural complications.[48] Furthermore, the CONFIRM registry evaluated procedural outcomes with OA in patients with CLI in 1109 patients (1544 lesions). Patients with below the knee lesions (BTK) had a higher incidence of perforation (1.5% vs 0.2%, $P = .005$), slow flow (7.7% vs 5.0%, $P = .03$), and spasm (10.3% vs 4.2%, $P<.001$) than patients treated above the knee. DE however was very low at 0.4% versus 5.1% for above the knee ($P<.001$).[36] Finally, given the low profile of the OA device, it is suitable for use from a transpedal approach (4-Fr profile and short 60-cm shaft option) for limb salvage in patients with severe calcified tibial disease.[49,50]

Directional Atherectomy

Zeller and colleagues[51] treated 36 limb ischemia patients (49 BTK lesions) with SilverHawk atherectomy. Average lesion length was 4.8 cm, and 22% were CTOs. Bailout stenting was needed in 4% of lesions because of dissection. Primary and secondary patency rates were 67% and 91% after 1 year, respectively. In addition, the

observational, nonrandomized, multicenter TALON registry[52] enrolled 601 consecutive patients (748 limbs, 1258 lesions) treated with the SilverHawk catheter. Mean lesion length below the knee was 3.3 cm. Procedural success was 97.6% with bailout stenting of 6.3% of lesions. TLR rate at 1 year in all lesions was 20% with no difference between diabetic and nondiabetic. There was a 3.3-fold increase in TLR rate in lesions longer than 100 mm. Furthermore, in the DEFINITIVE LE study,[53] of the 800 patients enrolled, 48.3% of patients had CLI and 68.3% were diabetics. CTO were 20.2% and mean lesion length was 5.8 cm. A high procedural success (less or equal 30%) was noted (84% of lesions). Also, the 1-year primary patency rate and freedom from major amputation were 78% and 93.1% in the CLI subgroup. Directional atherectomy with the SilverHawk device appears to be a viable option for treating infrapopliteal disease. In the authors' experience, it is most practical for short, focal lesions and mostly in the proximal and mid segments of the tibial and peroneal vessels.

Laser Atherectomy

Excimer laser is an effective device in infrapopliteal disease particularly suited for nonseverely calcified tibial and peroneal disease (Fig. 14). Given the availability of small catheter sizes (0.9 and 1.4 mm), the laser is capable of treating distal tibial and pedal arteries. Gray and colleagues[54] prospectively evaluated laser atherectomy (LA) in 23 patients (25 limbs) with CLI with infrainguinal disease (mixed inflow and outflow lesions). Procedural success was 88% with

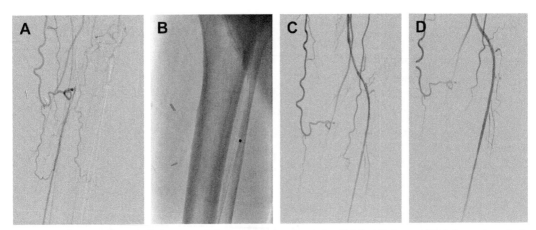

Fig. 14. LA for a totally occluded restenotic left popliteal and anterior tibialis (A). Laser elite 1.4 seen in anterior tibialis vessel (B). Postlaser (C). Postadjunctive angioplasty of the left anterior tibialis (D).

significant improvement in wound size and a high limb salvage rate. In addition, the Limb Salvage Following Laser-Assisted Angioplasty for Critical Limb Ischemia (LACI) Trial[55] enrolled 145 poor surgical patients for bypass surgery to receive LA. Most patients had advanced wounds and complex anatomic disease (90% CTO and 60% The Trans-Atlantic Inter-Society Consensus-D [TASC-D] lesions). Most patients received adjunctive PTA, and 45% of lesions were stented. Median lesion length was 11 cm. At 6 months, amputation rate was 7%. The LACI trial demonstrated the effectiveness and safety of the laser in advanced limb ischemia patients with advanced complex and poor outflow disease. Furthermore, in a retrospective study of 731 patients,[56] laser-assisted balloon angioplasty was compared with PTA alone in CLI patients with popliteal and infrapopliteal disease. There were more TASC-D lesions (92.5 vs 66.7%; P<.0001) and CTOs in the laser-assisted group. Multivariate analysis showed that the laser improved procedural success with an odds ratio (OR) of 7.59 to achieve less than 50% residual narrowing and OR of 4.77 to improve lesion severity score than PTA alone. At 36 months follow-up,[57] there were no differences in the need for repeat revascularization or major amputation in the 2 groups of patients despite the more complex disease in the laser arm. This study confirmed several prior observations that atherectomy does improve the acute procedural success of PTA and may offer some long-term advantages over PTA alone.

Rotational and JetStream Atherectomy

Data on rotational and JetStream atherectomy (JS) in infrapopliteal lesions are insufficient to make firm conclusions about the short- and long-term effectiveness of these devices in patients with limb ischemia. In the author's experience, both JetStream and rotational atherectomy are effective in treating calcified infrapopliteal disease. The JetStream is available as a single cutter with 2 sizes, 1.6 and 1.85. Superficial calcium removal has been demonstrated to occur effectively with JetStream,[30] and therefore, these 2 sizes are practical to use in proximal and mid tibial and peroneal vessels. Rotational atherectomy burrs are available in sizes 1.25 to 1.75 mm, which are suitable for infrapopliteal vessels. These burrs can be inserted via 5-Fr and 6-Fr sheaths. The disadvantage of rotational atherectomy in infrapopliteal calcified vessels is the need to use 0.009-inch wire and the potential need to upsize the burr.

ATHERECTOMY FOR IN-STENT RESTENOSIS

ISR following treatment of FP arteries occurs at an incidence of 19% to 37% per year and tends to be progressive for several years.[2–7] Treatment of restenotic lesions by PTA carries a high rate of recurrent restenosis and TLR.[58] Recently, LA,[59] covered stents,[60] and DCBs[61,62] were shown to be superior to PTA in treating ISR with a reduction in TLR and improved patency.

Directional Atherectomy with SilverHawk

SA is contraindicated in treating FP ISR in the United States because of potential cutter entrapment on stent struts. Small observational studies have shown however that this technique is effective in removing restenotic tissue with high procedural success.[63–65] The acute procedural success has been reported to be in the range of 97% to 100% with bailout stenting from 9% to 24%. The long-term results have varied in different studies with patency ranging from 25% to 49% and TLR rates from 31.7% to 47% at 1 to 2 years. It is also apparent that the higher patency and freedom from TLR rates at 6 months are not sustained with a rapid decline in patency and freedom from TLR between 6 months and 1 year.[64,65] The application of SA in treating FP ISR is associated with a high rate of DE reaching 80% to 85% of cases with over one/third of the debris being macrodebris.[64] DE requiring additional treatment ranged from 7.3% to 11% and was numerically higher in patients with no embolic filer protection. EFP is off label with the use of SA in FP ISR but may be an important tool to protect against significant DE. Finally, meticulous technique is needed with slow advancement of the cutter, frequent packing, and emptying of the nosecone, avoiding long cuts, and closely watching the relationship of the cutter to the stent under fluoroscopy.

JetStream Atherectomy

JS is currently an off-label application in FP ISR in the United States but recently received a Conformité Européene mark in Europe for this indication. JS was applied in a porcine stent/balloon overstretch injury model[66] and showed a significant tissue removal that was incremental by moving from a blade-down (BD) mode to a blade-up mode (BU). When each run is defined as a forward movement of the JS from proximal to distal end of the restenotic segment, 2 BD and 2 BU modes have shown by quantitative vascular angiography (QVA) and IVUS to yield maximum tissue removal. Also, scanning electron microscopy and high-dose radiographs did not demonstrate stent-device interaction with no stent deformity or strut discontinuation noted. Similarly, the same findings were seen in patients with ISR,[67] which also demonstrated an added gain in MLA following adjunctive PTA.

Clinical data on the JS in FP ISR are currently limited to small observational studies. Using the predecessor of JS, the Pathway device, Beschorner and colleagues[68] noted a 1-year primary patency rate of 33% in 33 patients treated for FP ISR. There were no device-related serious events. The JS version of the device has been markedly improved over the Pathway. JS has more powerful cutting ability, has more suction capacity, and yields larger MLA. Shammas and colleagues[32] have recently published their data from the prospective JetStream-ISR registry on 29 patients (32 limbs) with total lesion length of 17.4 ± 13.1 cm and total treated length 19.5 ± 12.9 cm. Acute procedural success (defined as <30% residual narrowing) was

100% (90.6% if defined with no adverse events), device success (defined as <50% residual with JS only) was 75.9%, and bailout stenting was 6.3% (excluding one stented case that was not a true bailout). DE requiring treatment occurred in 9.4% (total 3 cases; 2 occurred with no filter, 1 with the Spider FX filter and none with the Nav-6 filter). Core laboratory evaluation showed no new stent fractures or deformities, and the 6-month and 1-year follow-up TLR were 13.8% and 41.4% patients, respectively. Patency rate was 72% at 6 months.

Currently, the pivotal IDE JET-ISR trial (clinicaltrials.gov; NCT02730234) is ongoing to extend on the observations of the JetStream ISR. JET-ISR is a prospective, multicenter registry that will enroll 140 patients at a maximum of 14 sites in the United States.

Laser Atherectomy in Femoropopliteal In-Stent Restenosis

LA is currently the only approved procedure in the United States to treat FP ISR. Early data from 40 consecutive patients treated mostly with the laser Elite have shown that LA is feasible with high acute procedural success (92.5%), but the 1-year TLR was 48.7%.[69] In addition, and using the laser Booster, the PATENT multicenter registry (Photoablation Using the Turbo-Booster and Excimer Laser for In-Stent Restenosis Treatment)[70] enrolled 90 patients (mean lesion length 12.3 cm) and showed a high procedural success at 96.7% with 10% of patients having DE. Freedom from TLR was 64.4% at 1 year and primary patency was 37.8%. Furthermore, the multicenter randomized EXCITE ISR trial (EXCImer Laser Randomized Controlled Study for Treatment of FemoropopliTEal In-Stent Restenosis)[59] demonstrated that the laser increased the procedural success of the procedure over PTA alone and with less dissection and bailout stenting. In this study, 250 patients were randomized to LA and adjunctive PTA (n = 169) versus PTA alone (n = 81). Despite long lesions (average lesion length was 19.6 cm) and a high rate of total occlusions (30.5%), procedural success was higher with LA versus PTA (93.5% vs 82.7%; P = .01). Also, freedom from TLR was 73.5% versus 51.8% (P<.005) with LA versus PTA alone, respectively. Although the data were favorable at 6 months and continued to show superiority of the laser over PTA at 1 year, a sharp decline in freedom from TLR was seen at 1 year (TLR rate approximately 47% at 1 year). Finally, data from Armstrong and colleagues[71] have shown that at 2 years and in patients with total occlusions, TLR with the laser (43%) was not different from PTA (48%), whereas more favorable data with the laser were seen in shorter and nonocclusive lesions.

DE occurs also significantly with LA. In the DEEP EMBOLI registry[42] (including both FP ISR and de novo lesions), macrodebris was seen in 22.2% of filters in patients treated with the laser. Other studies have also shown that macrodebris was detected in 65.2% of filters when a filter is used in treating FP ISR with the laser.[69] DE requiring additional treatment ranged from 2.5% to 10%. Similarly to other atherectomy devices, a low threshold to use filters in treating FP ISR is recommended. Typically, these lesions are a mix of restentotic and thrombotic disease[72] with a high risk of embolic potential. A study comparing operators' choice in treating FP ISR between the laser and SA showed that the laser was preferred for longer (222 mm vs 114 mm) and more complex lesions (total occlusions 69% vs 20%).[73] This finding is likely driven by the user-friendly nature of the LA device when compared with SA in treating complex, long lesions.

Atherectomy with Adjunctive Antiproliferative Therapy

DCB and drug-coated stents have shown excellent results in treating short and noncomplex FP ISR lesions with patency ranging from 70.5% to 92.1% and TLR rates from 9.2% to 13.6% at 1 year.[61,62] Combining atherectomy and DCB is likely to be advantageous in more complex lesions, such as total occlusions and long lesions than DCB alone. Current data are limited to small observational studies showing patency rates of 84.7% to 91.7% at 9 months to 1 year and a TLR rate of 7% to 16.7%.[74–76] In one small randomized study that included 48 CLI patients with chronic SFA in-stent occlusions,[76] LA with DCB showed a superior patency (66.7% vs 37.5%), freedom from TLR (16.7% vs 50%), and lower amputation (8% vs 46%) rates at 1 year than DCB alone, respectively. Larger randomized data are needed to determine the true added advantage of atherectomy and DCB over DCB alone in patients with FP ISR.

In summary, atherectomy improves the acute procedural success of a procedure whether treating de novo or restenotic (including in-stent) disease. This higher procedural success is translated into lower residual stenosis, less dissection, and less bailout stenting. The intermediate follow-up results seem to be in favor of atherectomy in delaying and reducing the need for repeat revascularization in patients with FP ISR. Although the data are not conclusive for de novo disease, numerically, though not statistically, atherectomy seems to have favorable TLR rates on intermediate follow-up. However, as more is learned about atherectomy and how it affect restenosis, it seems that refining the technique and improving visualization during directional atherectomy may have an impact on reducing restenosis and TLR. Recent data suggest that avoiding cutting into the EEL is an important factor in reducing restenosis. The interplay between directional atherectomy and DCB is unclear. Could deeper cuts offset the benefit of DCB or could they actually allow deeper penetration of antiproliferative drugs and more effective DCB results? Would rotational atherectomy yield superior data with DCB than directional atherectomy given its differential cutting and avoiding deeper cuts? Would different DCB have different outcomes after atherectomy? We do not have answers to these questions, but certainly we are now capable of testing these hypotheses and more. The coming years will certainly yield valuable data and allow a more refined algorithm in treating de novo or restenotic disease in the infrainguinal arteries.

REFERENCES

1. Hong MS, Beck AW, Nelson PR. Emerging national trends in the management and outcomes of lower extremity peripheral arterial disease. Ann Vasc Surg 2011;25:44–54.
2. Laird JR, Katzen BT, Scheinert D, et al. Nitinol stent implantation versus balloon angioplasty for lesions in the superficial femoral artery and proximal popliteal artery: twelve-month results from the RESILIENT randomized trial. Circ Cardiovasc Interv 2010;3:267–76.
3. Krankenberg H, Schluter M, Steinkamp HJ, et al. Nitinol stent implantation versus percutaneous transluminal angioplasty in superficial femoral artery lesions up to 10 cm in length: the femoral artery stenting trial (FAST). Circulation 2007;116: 285–92.
4. Schillinger M, Sabeti S, Loewe C, et al. Balloon angioplasty versus implantation of nitinol stents in the superficial femoral artery. N Engl J Med 2006;354: 1879–88.
5. Dake MD, Ansel GM, Jaff MR, et al, Zilver PTX Investigators. Paclitaxel-eluting stents show superiority to balloon angioplasty and bare metal stents in femoropopliteal disease: twelve-month Zilver PTX randomized study results. Circ Cardiovasc Interv 2011;4:495–504.
6. Rastan A, Krankenberg H, Baumgartner I, et al. Stent placement versus balloon angioplasty for the treatment of obstructive lesions of the popliteal

artery: a prospective, multicenter, randomized trial. Circulation 2013;25(127):2535–41.

7. Laird JR. Limitations of percutaneous transluminal angioplasty and stenting for the treatment of disease of the superficial femoral and popliteal arteries. J Endovasc Ther 2006;13(Suppl 2):II30–40.

8. Shammas NW. An overview of optimal endovascular strategy in treating the femoropopliteal artery: mechanical, biological, and procedural factors. Int J Angiol 2013;22(1):1–8.

9. Zeller T. DEFINITIVE AR. Presented at VIVA 2014, Las Vegas (NE). Available at: http://evtoday.com/2014/10/covidien-presents-12-month-definitive-ar-results. Accessed December 30, 2016.

10. Scheller B, Speck U, Abramjuk C, et al. Paclitaxel balloon coating, a novel method for prevention and therapy of restenosis. Circulation 2004;110(7):810–4.

11. Scheinert D, Duda S, Zeller T, et al. The LEVANT I (Lutonix paclitaxel-coated balloon for the prevention of femoropopliteal restenosis) trial for femoropopliteal revascularization: first-in-human randomized trial of low-dose drug-coated balloon versus uncoated balloon angioplasty. JACC Cardiovasc Interv 2014;7(1):10–9.

12. Tepe G, Zeller T, Albrecht T, et al. Local delivery of paclitaxel to inhibit restenosis during angioplasty of the leg. N Engl J Med 2008;358:689–99.

13. Werk M, Albrecht T, Meyer DR, et al. Paclitaxel-coated balloons reduce restenosis after femoropopliteal angioplasty: evidence from the randomized PACIFIER trial. Circ Cardiovasc Interv 2012;5:831–40.

14. Werk M, Langner S, Reinkensmeier B, et al. Inhibition of restenosis in femoropopliteal arteries: paclitaxel-coated versus uncoated balloon: femoral paclitaxel randomized pilot trial. Circulation 2008;13:1358–65.

15. Liistro F, Grotti S, Porto I, et al. Drug-eluting balloon in peripheral intervention for the superficial femoral artery: the DEBATE-SFA randomized trial (drug eluting balloon in peripheral intervention for the superficial femoral artery). JACC Cardiovasc Interv 2013;6(12):1295–302.

16. Rosenfield K, Jaff MR, White CJ, et al, LEVANT 2 Investigators. Trial of a paclitaxel-coated balloon for femoropopliteal artery disease. N Engl J Med 2015;373:145–53.

17. Bishop PD, Feiten LE, Ouriel K, et al. Arterial calcification increases in distal arteries in patients with peripheral arterial disease. Ann Vasc Surg 2008; 22(6):799–805.

18. Rocha-Singh KJ, Zeller T, Jaff MR. Peripheral arterial calcification: prevalence, mechanism, detection, and clinical implications. Catheter Cardiovasc Interv 2014;83(6):E212–20.

19. Kashyap VS, Pavkov ML, Bishop PD, et al. Angiography underestimates peripheral atherosclerosis: lumenography revisited. J Endovasc Ther 2008; 15(1):117–25.

20. Shammas NW, Coiner D, Shammas G, et al. Predictors of provisional stenting in patients undergoing lower extremity arterial interventions. Int J Angiol 2011;20:95–100.

21. Fanelli F, Cannavale A, Gazzetti M, et al. Calcium burden assessment and impact on drug-eluting balloons in peripheral arterial disease. Cardiovasc Intervent Radiol 2014;37(4):898–907.

22. Tepe G, Beschorner U, Ruether C, et al. Drug-eluting balloon therapy for femoropopliteal occlusive disease: predictors of outcome with a special emphasis on Calcium. J Endovasc Ther 2015;22(5): 727–33.

23. Hwang CW, Levin AD, Jonas M, et al. Thrombosis modulates arterial drug distribution for drug-eluting stents. Circulation 2005;111(13):1619–26.

24. Shammas NW, Coiner D, Shammas GA, et al. Percutaneous lower-extremity arterial interventions with primary balloon angioplasty versus Silverhawk atherectomy and adjunctive balloon angioplasty: randomized trial. J Vasc Interv Radiol 2011;22(9): 1223–8.

25. Shammas NW, Lam R, Mustapha J, et al. Comparison of orbital atherectomy plus balloon angioplasty vs. balloon angioplasty alone in patients with critical limb ischemia: results of the CALCIUM 360 randomized pilot trial. J Endovasc Ther 2012; 19(4):480–8.

26. Dattilo R, Himmelstein SI, Cuff RF. The COMPLIANCE 360° Trial: a randomized, prospective, multicenter, pilot study comparing acute and long-term results of orbital atherectomy to balloon angioplasty for calcified femoropopliteal disease. J Invasive Cardiol 2014;26(8):355–60.

27. Tzafriri AR, Nikanorov A, Zani B, et al. TCT-794. Lesion preparation with an orbital atherectomy system enhances paclitaxel deposition in calcified peripheral arteries. J Am Coll Cardiol 2015;66(15 Suppl B):B323.

28. Shammas NW. An algorithm-based approach to optimize endovascular outcomes of complex infrainguinal peripheral arterial disease. Vasc Dis Management 2016;13(6):E128–36.

29. Shammas NW. JETSTREAM atherectomy: a review of technique, tips, and tricks in treating the femoropopliteal lesions. Int J Angiol 2015;24:81–6.

30. Maehara A, Mintz GS, Shimshak TM, et al. Intravascular ultrasound evaluation of JETSTREAM atherectomy removal of superficial calcium in peripheral arteries. EuroIntervention 2015;11(1):96–103.

31. Banerjee A, Sarode K, Mohammad A, et al. Safety and effectiveness of the Nav-6 filter in preventing distal embolization during Jetstream atherectomy of infrainguinal peripheral artery lesions. J Invasive Cardiol 2016;28:330–3.

32. Shammas NW, Shammas GA, Banerjee S, et al. JetStream rotational and aspiration atherectomy in

treating in-stent restenosis of the femoropopliteal arteries: results of the JETSTREAM-ISR Feasibility Study. J Endovasc Ther 2016;23:339–46.

33. Zeller T, Krankenberg H, Steinkamp H, et al. One-year outcome of percutaneous rotational atherectomy with aspiration in infrainguinal peripheral arterial occlusive disease: the multicenter pathway PVD trial. J Endovasc Ther 2009;16:653–62.

34. Shammas NW, Gray W, Garcia L, et al. Preliminary results from the Jetstream navitus system Endovascular Therapy post-market (JET) registry. J Am Coll Cardiol 2013;62(Suppl 1):B163.

35. Das T, Mustapha J, Indes J, et al. Technique optimization of orbital atherectomy in calcified peripheral lesions of the lower extremities: the CONFIRM series, a prospective multicenter registry. Catheter Cardiovasc Interv 2014;83:115–22.

36. Lee MS, Mustapha J, Beasley R, et al. Impact of lesion location on procedural and acute angiographic outcomes in patients with critical limb ischemia treated for peripheral artery disease with orbital atherectomy: a CONFIRM registries subanalysis. Catheter Cardiovasc Interv 2016;87:440–5.

37. Weinstock B, Dattilo R, Diage T. Cost-effectiveness analysis of orbital atherectomy plus balloon angioplasty vs balloon angioplasty alone in subjects with calcified femoropopliteal lesions. Clinicoecon Outcomes Res 2014;6:133–9.

38. Roberts D, Niazi K, Miller W, et al, DEFINITIVE Ca^{++} Investigators. Effective endovascular treatment of calcified femoropopliteal disease with directional atherectomy and distal embolic protection: final results of the DEFINITIVE Ca^{++} trial. Catheter Cardiovasc Interv 2014;84(2):236–44.

39. McKinsey JF, Zeller T, Rocha-Singh KJ, et al, DEFINITIVE LE Investigators. Lower extremity revascularization using directional atherectomy: 12-month prospective results of the DEFINITIVE LE study. JACC Cardiovasc Interv 2014;7(8):923–33.

40. VISION trial. Available at: http://www.invasive-cardiology.com/news/avingers-pantheris-image-guided-atherectomy-system-receives-fda-510k-clearance-pad. Accessed December 30, 2016.

41. Cioppa A, Stabile E, Popusoi G, et al. Combined treatment of heavy calcified femoro-popliteal lesions using directional atherectomy and a paclitaxel coated balloon: one-year single centre clinical results. Cardiovasc Revasc Med 2012;13(4):219–23.

42. Shammas NW, Coiner D, Shammas GA, et al. Distal embolic event protection using excimer laser ablation in peripheral vascular interventions: results of the DEEP EMBOLI registry. J Endovasc Ther 2009;16:197–202.

43. Lam RC, Shah S, Faried PL, et al. Incidence and clinical significance of distal embolization during percutaneous interventions involving the superficial femoral artery. J Vasc Surg 2007;46:1155–9.

44. Dave RM, Patlola R, Kollmeyer K, et al, CELLO Investigators. Excimer laser recanalization of femoropopliteal lesions and 1-year patency: results of the CELLO registry. J Endovasc Ther 2009;16:665–75.

45. Scheinert D, Laird JR, Schroder M, et al. Excimer laser-assisted recanalization of long, chronic superficial femoral artery occlusions. J Endovasc Ther 2001;8:156–66.

46. Laird JR. Peripheral excimer laser angioplasty (PELA) trial results. Presentation at Late Breaking Trials. Transcatheter Cardiovascular Therapeutics Annual Meeting. Washington, DC, September 24–28, 2002.

47. Safian RD, Niazi K, Runyon JP, et al, OASIS Investigators. Orbital atherectomy for infrapopliteal disease: device concept and outcome data for the OASIS trial. Catheter Cardiovasc Interv 2009;73:406–12.

48. Panaich SS, Arora S, Patel N, et al. In-hospital outcomes of atherectomy during endovascular lower extremity revascularization. Am J Cardiol 2016;117:676–84.

49. Mustapha JA, Saab F, McGoff T, et al. TAMI technique: tibiopedal arterial minimally invasive retrograde revascularization. Endovascular Today 2013;1:39–47.

50. Wu W, Moore K, Wu A, et al. The transpedal approach for peripheral intervention: innovative or alternative? Is transpedal access the future of peripheral revascularization? Endovascular Today 2015;48–53.

51. Zeller T, Sixt S, Schwarzwälder U, et al. Two-year results after directional atherectomy of infrapopliteal arteries with the SilverHawk device. J Endovasc Ther 2007;14:232–40.

52. Ramaiah V, Gammon R, Kiesz S, et al, TALON Registry. Midterm outcomes from the TALON Registry: treating peripherals with SilverHawk: outcomes collection. J Endovasc Ther 2006;13:592–602.

53. Rastan A, McKinsey JF, Garcia LA, et al, DEFINITIVE LE Investigators. One-year outcomes following directional atherectomy of infrapopliteal artery lesions: subgroup results of the prospective, multicenter DEFINITIVE LE Trial. J Endovasc Ther 2015;22:839–46.

54. Gray BH, Laird JR, Ansel GM, et al. Complex endovascular treatment for critical limb ischemia in poor surgical candidates: a pilot study. J Endovasc Ther 2002;9:599–604.

55. Laird JR, Zeller T, Gray BH, et al, LACI Investigators. Limb salvage following laser-assisted angioplasty for critical limb ischemia: results of the LACI multicenter trial. J Endovasc Ther 2006;13:1–11.

56. Singh T, Kodenchery M, Artham S, et al. Laser in infrapopliteal and popliteal stenosis (LIPS): retrospective review of laser-assisted balloon angioplasty versus balloon angioplasty alone for below

knee arterial disease. Cardiovasc Interven Ther 2014;29:109–16.

57. Piyaskulkaew C, Parvataneni K, Ballout H, et al. Laser in infrapopliteal and popliteal stenosis 2 study (LIPS2): long-term outcomes of laser-assisted balloon angioplasty versus balloon angioplasty for below knee peripheral arterial disease. Catheter Cardiovasc Interv 2015;86:1211–8.

58. Shammas NW, Jones-Miller S, Lemke J. Meta-analysis-derived benchmarks of patency and target lesion revascularization of percutaneous balloon angioplasty from prospective clinical trials of symptomatic femoropopliteal in-stent restenosis. J Vasc Interv Radiol 2016;27:1195–203.

59. Dippel EJ, Makam P, Kovach R, et al. Randomized controlled study of excimer laser atherectomy for treatment of femoropopliteal in-stent restenosis: initial results from the EXCITE ISR trial (EXCImer Laser Randomized Controlled Study for Treatment of FemoropopliTEal In-Stent Restenosis). JACC Cardiovasc Interv 2015;8(1 Pt A):92–101.

60. Bosiers M, Deloose K, Callaert J, et al. Superiority of stent-grafts for in-stent restenosis in the superficial femoral artery: twelve-month results from a multicenter randomized trial. J Endovasc Ther 2015;22:1–10.

61. Krankenberg H, Tübler T, Ingwersen M, et al. Drug-coated balloon versus standard balloon for superficial femoral artery in-stent restenosis: the Randomized Femoral Artery In-Stent Restenosis (FAIR) Trial. Circulation 2015;132(23):2230–6.

62. Kinstner CM, Lammer J, Willfort-Ehringer A, et al. Paclitaxel-eluting balloon versus standard balloon angioplasty in in-stent restenosis of the superficial femoral and proximal popliteal artery: 1-year results of the PACUBA Trial. JACC Cardiovasc Interv 2016;9:1386–92.

63. Trentmann J, Charalambous N, Djawanscher M, et al. Safety and efficacy of directional atherectomy for the treatment of in-stent restenosis of the femoropopliteal artery. Cardiovasc Surg (Torino) 2010; 51(4):551–60.

64. Shammas NW, Shammas GA, Helou TJ, et al. Safety and 1-year revascularization outcome of SilverHawk atherectomy in treating in-stent restenosis of femoropopliteal arteries: A retrospective review from a single center. Cardiovasc Revasc Med 2012;13:341–4.

65. Brodmann M, Rief P, Froehlich H, et al. Neointimal hyperplasia after Silverhawk atherectomy versus percutaneous transluminal angioplasty (PTA) in femoropopliteal stent reobstructions: a controlled, randomized pilot trial. Cardiovasc Intervent Radiol 2013;36:69–74.

66. Shammas NW, Aasen N, Bailey L, et al. Two blades-up runs using the Jetstream navitus atherectomy device achieve optimal tissue debulking of nonocclusive in-stent restenosis: observations from a porcine stent/balloon injury model. J Endovasc Ther 2015;22(4):518–24.

67. Shammas NW, Shammas GA, Aasen N, et al. Number of blades-up runs using Jetstream XC atherectomy for optimal tissue debulking in patients with femoropopliteal artery in-stent restenosis. J Vasc Interv Radiol 2015;26(12):1847–51.

68. Beschorner U, Krankenberg H, Scheinert D, et al. Rotational and aspiration atherectomy for infrainguinal in-stent restenosis. Vasa 2013;42:127–33.

69. Shammas NW, Shammas GA, Hafez A, et al. Safety and one-year revascularization outcome of excimer laser ablation therapy in treating in-stent restenosis of femoropopliteal arteries: a retrospective review from a single center. Cardiovasc Revasc Med 2012;13(6):341–4.

70. Schmidt A, Zeller T, Sievert H, et al. Photoablation using the turbo-booster and excimer laser for in-stent restenosis treatment: twelve-month results from the PATENT study. J Endovasc Ther 2014;21:52–60.

71. Armstrong EJ, Thiruvoipati T, Tanganyika K, et al. Laser atherectomy for treatment of femoropopliteal in-stent restenosis. J Endovasc Ther 2015;22: 506–13.

72. Shammas NW, Dippel EJ, Shammas G, et al. Dethrombosis of the lower extremity arteries using the power-pulse spray technique in patients with recent onset thrombotic occlusions: results of the DETHROMBOSIS Registry. J Endovasc Ther 2008; 15:570–9.

73. Shammas NW, Shammas GA, Jerin M. Differences in patient selection and outcomes between SilverHawk atherectomy and laser ablation in the treatment of femoropopliteal in-stent restenosis: a retrospective analysis from a single center. J Endovasc Ther 2013;20:844–52.

74. van den Berg JC, Pedrotti M, Canevascini R, et al. In-stent restenosis: mid-term results of debulking using excimer laser and drug-eluting balloons: sustained benefit? J Invasive Cardiol 2014;26:333–7.

75. Sixt S, Carpio Cancino OG, Treszl A, et al. Drug-coated balloon angioplasty after directional atherectomy improves outcome in restenotic femoropopliteal arteries. J Vasc Surg 2013;58:682–6.

76. Gandini R, Del Giudice C, Merolla S, et al. Treatment of chronic SFA in-stent occlusion with combined laser atherectomy and drug-eluting balloon angioplasty in patients with critical limb ischemia: a single-center, prospective, randomized study. J Endovasc Ther 2013;20:805–14.

Contemporary Outcomes of Endovascular Intervention for Critical Limb Ischemia

Pratik K. Dalal, MD, Anand Prasad, MD, FSCAI, RPVI*

KEYWORDS

- Critical limb ischemia • Peripheral arterial disease • Revascularization

---

KEY POINTS

- Critical limb ischemia (CLI) remains an important cause of significant morbidity and mortality.
- Although limited randomized data are available, an endovascular first approach seems an acceptable alternative to open surgery, especially in patients with high risk of morbidity and mortality in the perioperative setting.
- Specific outcomes in the CLI population vary among trials related to a variety of endovascular therapies, patient populations, and inconsistent administration and reporting of adjunctive wound care.
- Newer therapeutic options for endovascular therapies, such as atherectomy devices and drug-coated balloons (DCBs), may improve procedural outcomes and durability but remain to be rigorously studied in the CLI population.

INTRODUCTION

It is estimated that more than 200 million people worldwide have lower extremity peripheral arterial disease (PAD).[1] Although the economic impact of symptomatic PAD is substantial, the morbidity and mortality in patients with CLI highlight the importance of this disease process. Modern data suggest that amputation rates of 35% to 67% persist in CLI patients.[2] The mortality after a first lower extremity amputation is estimated to be 25% at 30 days and 50% at 1 year.[3] The cause of death in the majority of these patients is related to cardiovascular causes — and as such CLI represents a potent marker for future cardiovascular risk.[4] Concordant with this statement are the recent data related to CLI admissions from the National Inpatient Sample, which demonstrated a steady decrease over the past decade in amputation rates in this population with a much less robust decline in mortality.[5]

TREATMENT STRATEGIES FOR CRITICAL LIMB ISCHEMIA

Given that CLI represents a marker for systemic vascular and often multisystem organ dysfunction (eg, renal disease, diabetes, and obesity), a 2-pronged approach addressing both limb salvage and the underlying medical comorbidities is obligatory. Although this review focuses on revascularization — specifically, the outcomes of endovascular therapy — the importance of medical therapy for reduction of future cardiovascular events should not be ignored. With regard to limb salvage, treatment of CLI is aimed at improving peripheral arterial perfusion via timely

---

Disclosure Statement: Dr A. Prasad reports research funding from Osprey Medical and Medtronic and speaking honoraria from Osprey Medical, AstraZeneca, Abiomed, and Gilead.
Department of Cardiovascular Diseases, University of Texas Health Science Center, 7703 Floyd Curl Drive, MC 7872, San Antonio, TX 78229, USA
* Corresponding author.
E-mail address: Prasada@uthscsa.edu

Intervent Cardiol Clin 6 (2017) 251–259
http://dx.doi.org/10.1016/j.iccl.2016.12.008

revascularization coupled with adjunctive wound care.

Antiplatelet Therapy

In patients with symptomatic PAD, antiplatelet therapy with aspirin alone or clopidogrel alone remains a class I recommendation.[6] Antiplatelet therapy confers a 22% odds reduction for cardiovascular events, including myocardial infarction, stroke, and vascular death.[7] Some data highlight the uncertainty in this field, however: a meta-analysis of 18 randomized controlled trials with more than 5200 patients did not find a statistically significant reduction in the primary endpoint of cardiovascular death, MI, and stroke.[8] Specific agents remain an active area of interest with clopidogrel demonstrated superior to aspirin in cardiovascular risk reduction in a population of patients with systemic atherosclerotic vascular disease, including symptomatic PAD.[9] Ticagrelor, a reversible inhibitor of P2Y12, was not shown superior to clopidogrel for the reduction of cardiovascular events in patients with symptomatic PAD.[10]

Vorapaxar is a novel antiplatelet agent that antagonizes the protease-activated receptor (PAR-1). By inhibition of PAR-1, thrombin-mediated platelet aggregation is inhibited. This receptor is also present on vascular endothelium and smooth muscle, where its mechanism of action result in mitogenicity.[11] Vorapaxar was found to reduce the incidence of cardiovascular death or ischemic events when added to a background of aspirin and thienopyrdine or warfarin in patients with a history of myocardial infarction, stroke, or peripheral vascular disease. There was an increased risk of bleeding, however, especially in patients with a history of stroke.[12] A prespecified PAD cohort containing more than 3500 patients with a history of intermittent claudication and ankle-brachial index less than 0.85 or previous revascularization for limb ischemia was also analyzed with respect to a composite endpoint of MI, stroke, and cardiovascular death and secondary endpoints of acute limb ischemia, peripheral revascularization (urgent and elective), and urgent hospitalization for vascular cause of an ischemic nature.[13] Vorapaxar did not reduce the risk of cardiovascular death, MI, or stroke in patients with PAD; however, vorapaxar significantly reduced acute limb ischemia and peripheral revascularization. These benefits were accompanied by a higher risk of bleeding. In the 2016 American Heart Association/American College of Cardiology Guideline on the Management of Patients with Lower Extremity Peripheral Artery Disease, vorapaxar has a class IIB (level of evidence B-R) indication for the medical management of PAD.[6]

Statin Therapy

In the Heart Protection Study, which included 6748 patients with PAD, 40 mg of simvastatin daily reduced the rate of first major vascular event by 22% relative to placebo.[14] Kumbhani and colleagues[15] showed that statin use in patients with PAD reduced 4-year adverse limb-related events (worsening claudication, new CLI, new lower extremity revascularization, and new ischemic amputation) compared with no statin use.

Angiotensin-converting Enzyme Inhibition

Angiotensin-converting enzyme inhibitors are currently a class IIA recommendation in the management of patients with PAD.[6] In patients who were normotensive at the time of enrollment, 4051 patients with PAD treated with ramipril experiences a 25% reduced risk of MI, stroke, or vascular death.[16]

Smoking Cessation

Perhaps the most critical intervention in the management of PAD is tobacco cessation counseling. Observational studies suggest that smoking cessation is associated with lower rates of cardiovascular ischemic events, limb-related events, bypass graft failure, amputation, and death in patients with PAD.[6,17–20]

Revascularization

The choice of revascularization approach has important implications in selecting endpoints and outcomes when performing trials for CLI patients. In the coronary literature, selecting between medical therapy, surgical bypass, or percutaneous coronary revascularization for individual patients has remained a moving target — with approximately 3 decades of randomized clinical trials. In contrast, there is a paucity of data to guide therapy in CLI. Prior to the development of endovascular techniques, open surgical approaches dominated the treatment of CLI. Limitations of surgery have centered on perioperative morbidity and mortality in a sick population and anatomic challenges related to adequate graft conduits, inadequate distal targets, and poor outflow. In part due to reduced procedural morbidity and mortality, endovascular techniques have become the first-line approach to CLI revascularization, with a marked temporal decline in surgical procedures.[5] This shift has been related to decreasing rates of major amputations in the United States — however, whether this relationship is causative or associative remains a point of uncertainty.

The early experience with balloon angioplasty compared with surgical revascularization in the

Bypass versus Angioplasty in Severe Ischemia of the Leg (BASIL): multicentre, randomised controlled trial demonstrated comparable amputation-free survival with surgery compared with an endovascular approach — with an associated higher perioperative morbidity and mortality in surgical patients (**Figs. 1** and **2**).[21] Since publication of BASIL, endovascular techniques and technology have rapidly expanded. Mechanisms to improve vessel patency now include various DCBs; drug-eluting stents (DESs); rotational, laser, and directional atherectomy; devices for crossing chronic total occlusions; true lumen re-entry devices; and embolic protection devices. The efficacy of these percutaneous therapies for CLI have been variable and largely derived from single-arm or nonrandomized studies. Novel techniques, such as retrograde pedal access and subintimal angioplasty, have broadened the lesion subsets approached by operators — challenging the traditional limitations of endovascular therapy, including long lesions, chronic total occlusions, and calcified vessels. Although the outcomes of individual approaches have rarely been vetted in a randomized fashion, the overall outcomes of open surgery versus contemporary endovascular therapy will be tested in the ongoing best endovascular versus best surgical therapy for patients with critical limb ischemia (BEST-CLI) trial.[22] The remaining focus of this review is on highlighting the outcomes of individual endovascular therapies for CLI, outlining the strengths and weaknesses based on published data.

DRUG-COATED BALLOONS

DCBs combine angioplasty with the delivery of an antiproliferative agent to the vessel wall in an effort to prevent restenosis. The potential of DCB use in CLI stems from their success in the femoropopliteal circulation. The data on outcomes of DCBs for treatment of infrapopliteal disease and CLI, however, have been mixed. The Drug-Coated Balloon versus Standard Percutaneous Transluminal Angioplasty for the Treatment of Superficial Femoral and/or Popliteal Peripheral Artery Disease (IN.PACT SFA) trial compared paclitaxel DCB to standard percutaneous transluminal angioplasty (PTA) in 331 patients with superficial femoral artery/popliteal disease.[23] DCB resulted in higher primary patency versus PTA (82.2% vs 52.4%; P<.001). The rate of clinically driven target lesion revascularization (TLR) was 2.4% in the DCB arm compared with 20.6% in the PTA arm (P<.001).

The Drug-Eluting Balloon in Peripheral Intervention for Below the Knee Angioplasty Evaluation (DEBATE-BTK) compared the performance of a novel DCB (IN.PACT Amphirion, Medtronic, Santa Rosa, California) with conventional PTA (1:1 randomization).[24] The study was performed in 158 diabetics with de novo, long lesions (78% CTOs) below the knee area using 1-year binary restenosis rate as the primary endpoint. Mean length of the treated segments was 129 mm ± 83 mm in the DCB group compared with 131 mm ± 79 mm in the PTA group (P = .7). At 1 year, the DCB group had a lower rate of restenosis (27% vs 74%, respectively; P<.001) and TLR (18% vs 43%, respectively; P = .01). There was no increase in amputations noted in the DCB arm.

The IN.PACT DEEP-Drug-eluting balloon versus standard balloon angioplasty for infrapopliteal arterial revascularization in critical limb ischemia: 12-month results from the IN.PACT DEEP randomized trial compared DCB versus standard PTA for infrapopliteal arterial revascularization in CLI.[25] This was a larger prospective, multicenter, randomized controlled trial with 358 CLI patients were randomized 2:1 to Amphirion DCBs or PTA. The primary efficacy endpoints

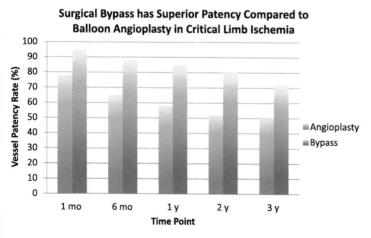

Surgical Bypass has Superior Patency Compared to Balloon Angioplasty in Critical Limb Ischemia

■ Angioplasty
■ Bypass

Fig. 1. Meta-analysis of infrapopliteal angioplasty versus surgery for chronic CLI (P<.05 across time points). (*Data from* Romiti M, Albers M, Brochado-Neto FC, et al. Meta-analysis of infrapopliteal angioplasty for chronic critical limb ischemia. J Vasc Surg 2008;47:975–81.)

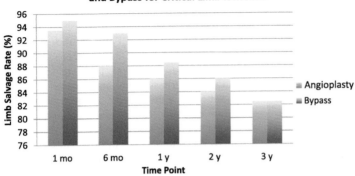

Limb Salvage Rates are Comparable Between Angioplasty and Bypass for Critical Limb Ischemia

Fig. 2. Meta-analysis of infrapopliteal angioplasty for chronic CLI (*P* = NS). NS, not significant. (*Data from* Romiti M, Albers M, Brochado-Neto FC, et al. Meta-analysis of infrapopliteal angioplasty for chronic critical limb ischemia. J Vasc Surg 2008; 47:975–81.)

were clinically driven TLR (CD-TLR) and late lumen loss assessed by an independent core laboratory. There was no difference between DCB and PTA in the primary efficacy endpoint (DCB vs PTA, respectively: clinically driven TLR of 9.2% vs 13.1% [*P* = .291] and late lumen loss of 0.61 mm ± 0.78 mm versus 0.62 mm ± 0.78 mm [*P* = .950]). Major amputation–free survival rates at 12 months were 81.1% and 89.2% (*P* = .057), respectively, in the DCB and PTA arms. The lack of efficacy and the numerically higher (but statistically nonsignificant) rate of amputations in the DCB arm raised concerns about the utility of this technology below the knee. The smaller trials that preceded IN.PACT DEEP were promising but were largely single center and lacked independent core laboratory adjudication. Despite a larger sample size, IN.PACT DEEP was small and had a high rate of loss to angiographic follow-up. Adjunctive therapy (wound care, débridement, antibiotics, and hyperbaric oxygen) all play an important role in successful healing and

these parameters were not controlled in the trial — an issue with many CLI studies (**Fig. 3**).

Several studies are re-evaluating the use of DCBs for treatment of infrapopliteal disease. The ongoing Lutonix Drug Coated Balloon versus Standard Balloon Angioplasty for Treatment of Below-the-Knee Arteries (LUTONIX BTK) trial (NCT01870401) will enroll 480 patients with CLI to examine the role of DCB therapy in infrapopliteal disease whereas the ongoing Atherectomy and Drug-Coated Balloon Angioplasty in Treatment of Long Infrapopliteal Lesions (ADCAT) study (NCT01763476) will investigate the role of atherectomy in conjunction with DCBs in below-the-knee disease.

STENTS

The Achilles heel of angioplasty has always been limitations in acute gain due to vessel recoil and dissection, coupled with neointimal proliferation and subsequent restenosis. The use of nitinol

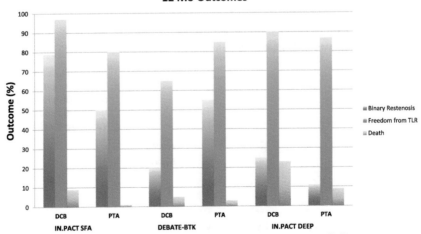

Fig. 3. Outcomes with DCBs versus standard angioplasty in CLI. *Data from* Refs.[20–22]

self-expanding stent technology has been commonplace in the superficial femoral artery and has shown improved patency versus PTA alone.[26] Limited options have existed for small diameter self-expanding stents below the knee, and off-label use of coronary stents in this circulation is well described.[27] The Xpert Nitinol Stenting for Critically Ischemic Lower Limbs (XCELL) trial evaluated safety and effectiveness of the Xpert self-expanding nitinol stent (Abbott Vascular, Redwood City, California) in Rutherford classes 4 to 6 CLI patients undergoing primary infrapopliteal stent deployment.[28] The study was a prospective, nonrandomized, multi-center, single-arm study with clinical follow-up at 1 month, 3 months, 6 months, and 12 months.[23] Despite a 6-month binary restenosis rate of 68.5%, the TLR was 29.9%. Twelve-month amputation-free survival was 78.3%; 62% of observable wounds had healed.

Balloon-expandable DESs have been compared with PTA (A Prospective Randomized Multicenter Comparison of Balloon Angioplasty and Infrapopliteal Stenting with the Sirolimus-Eluting Stent in Patients with Ischemic Peripheral Arterial Disease [ACHILLES]) and randomized comparison of everolimus-eluting versus bare-metal stents in patients with critical limb ischemia and infrapopliteal arterial occlusive disease (DESTINY) and Sirolimus-eluting stents versus bare-metal stents for treatment of focal lesions in infrapopliteal arteries: a double-blind, multi-centre, randomized clinical trial (YUKON-BTK).[29] Specific drug therapy (paclitaxel vs sirolimus) was compared in the Preventing Amputations using Drug eluting Stents (PaRADISE) trial in patients with CLI.[27] These studies have all been limited by small sample sizes and variable comparator groups. For example, the PaRADISE study data were nonrandomized and compared outcomes to historic data from the Trans-Atlantic Inter-Society Consensus for the Management of Peripheral Arterial Disease (TASC II) document and level 1 evidence from the BASIL trial to account for a lack of a control arm. The PaRADISE study 1-year and 3-year freedom from major amputation rates were 96% and 94%, respectively, and at 3 years the PaRADISE study maintained a 13% ± 6.3% limb survival advantage over the BASIL trial (**Fig. 4**).[27]

Fusaro and colleagues[30] performed an updated meta-analysis of DESs for infrapopliteal arteries, which included 611 patients from 5 trials. The key findings of the analysis are a median lesion length of 26.8 mm (range: 18.2–30.0 mm) and median reference vessel diameter of 2.86 mm (range: 2.68–3.00 mm). At a median follow-up of 12 months, DESs reduced the risk of TLR ($P < .001$), restenosis ($P < .001$), and amputation ($P = .04$). Despite the favorable results, these findings may not be applicable to many real-world patients given the short lesion lengths and large reference diameters.

More recently, the Absorb bioresorbable vascular scaffold (Abbott Vascular, Santa Clara, California) has been evaluated in the infrapopliteal circulation.[31] The resorbable nature of the device gives it significant potential for positive blood vessel wall remodeling, stabilization of the atheromatous plaque, and potential return of endothelial function. Patients were considered suitable for treatment with a bioresorbable vascular scaffold if they had Rutherford-Becker class 3 to 6 symptoms from de novo stenotic lesions greater than 60% of the tibial or distal popliteal arteries with length less than or equal to 5 cm and vessel diameters of 2.5 mm to 4.0 mm in which significant inflow stenoses had been successfully treated and if they had at least 1 single-vessel outflow to the foot. The primary

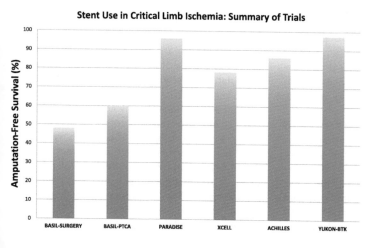

Stent Use in Critical Limb Ischemia: Summary of Trials

Fig. 4. Amputation-free survival with stents in below-the-knee interventions. XCELL, Major Adverse Limb Events and Wound Healing Following Infrapopliteal Artery Stent Implantation in Patients with Critical Limb Ischemia. *Data from* Refs.[18,24–27]

endpoint was freedom from binary restenosis. Color-flow Doppler was used to assess the scaffold for restenotic endpoints. The mean duration of follow-up was 12.0 months ± 3.9 months. At ultrasound follow-up, 3 of 50 scaffolds (6%) patent on hospital discharge had developed binary restenosis. Freedom from clinically driven TLR was estimated at 96.0% at 6 months, 12 months, and 24 months by the Kaplan-Meier method. The primary patency rate was 96.0% at 6 months, 96.0% at 12 months, and 84.6% at 24 months. On the basis of wound status and patient symptoms, 30 of 38 limbs (79%) had improved clinically, 7 (18%) were unchanged, and 1 (2.6%) was worse. Although the results are encouraging, much like the early DES trials, larger randomized data are needed with this technology.

ATHERECTOMY

Driven by advancements in technology and a favorable reimbursement paradigm in the United States, the use of atherectomy has increased in the past decade.[32,33] Despite this increased utilization, routine use of atherectomy compared with PTA alone or in combination with stenting has not been rigorously studied in a randomized fashion. Multiple studies, however, have demonstrated the use of atherectomy with adjunctive PTA in the context of infrapopliteal disease — particularly when calcium is involved in vessel pathology.[34]

Grouping atherectomy devices into a single term is misleading because laser, orbital, and rotational debulking and plaque modification all use different methods, carry unique risks, and result in variable luminal gain. The outcomes of specific devices have also lacked direct head-to-head comparisons in a randomized fashion. In a series of 418 patients undergoing tibial intervention (333 PTA and 79 atherectomy), Todd and colleagues[35] noted no differences in primary or secondary patency, limb salvage, or overall survival between the treatment groups. The cost of the devices (often more than $2000) coupled with the potential for distal embolization and concomitant need for embolic protection devices has been an ongoing area of investigation and controversy.

Laird and colleagues[36] evaluated the use of laser-assisted angioplasty for CLI among patients who were poor candidates for surgical revascularization. Endovascular treatment included guide wire traversal and excimer laser angioplasty followed by PTA with optional stenting. This trial enrolled 145 patients with 155 critically ischemic limbs in a multicenter, nonrandomized fashion. Procedural success, defined as less than 50% residual stenosis in all treated lesions, was seen in 86% of limbs. Stents were implanted in 45% of limbs. At 6-month follow-up, limb salvage was achieved in 110 (92%) of 119 surviving patients or 118 (93%) 127 limbs.

Lower extremity directional atherectomy (Medtronic) was studied in the Determination of Effectiveness of the SilverHawk (®) Peripheral Plaque Excision Systems (SilverHawk Device Medtronic) for the Treatment of Infrainguinal Vessels/Lower Extremities (DEFINITIVE LE) trial.[37] DEFINITIVE LE claudicants with infrapopliteal lesions had a 5.5-cm mean lesion length and a 90% primary patency rate; CLI subjects had a 6.0-cm mean lesion length, a 78% primary patency rate, and a 95% limb salvage rate. The longer lesions in the infrapopliteal arteries, regardless of diabetic status, showed better patency outcomes than similar length lesions in the SFA and popliteal arteries. The DEFINITIVE LE study demonstrated that directional atherectomy is a safe and effective treatment modality at 12 months for a diverse patient population with either claudication or CLI. The limb salvage rate of 95% observed in the DEFINITIVE LE CLI cohort is higher than the referenced CLI surgical bypass studies that reported rates between 81% and 87%.

Rotational atherectomy with the Rotablator system (Boston Scientific, Marlborough, MA) has been extensively used in the coronary circulation — and the utility of this technology in the peripheral arterial bed was first described approximately 2 decades ago. The initial experiences were variable with not infrequent complications in 31 of 72 patients (13% hemoglobinuria, 10% emboli, 6% dissections, 4% perforations, 5% hematoma, and 1% infection)[38]; 11% of patients also had early thrombosis. Technique, operator familiarity, and availability of more potent antiplatelet therapy have made rotablation therapy in the coronary — and potentially in the peripheral — bed safer. This remains speculative, however, because a large contemporary data set on Rotablator outcomes in CLI is not available. The mechanism of Rotablator therapy involving differential ablation and luminal gain certainly lends itself to promise in calcified tibial vessels — which are often comparable to size proximally to coronary vessels.

More recent rotational tools, such as the Jetstream rotational atherectomy system (Boston Scientific) and the Phoenix device (Volcano, San Diego, CA), introduce mechanisms to limit distal embolization. The Jetstream catheter provides active aspiration with rotational atherectomy with or without simultaneous blade based plaque cutting. The Phoenix catheter system uses an automated Archimedes screw design to actively debulk and then bring plaque back into a waste bag. Whether these technologies limit distal embolization remains uncertain; however, some data suggest low rates of this complication.

The largest bulk of data for outcomes using the most recent iterations of the Jetstream system are focused on femoropopliteal lesions with a paucity of CLI patients.[39,40] The Phoenix catheter was studied in a single-arm, multicenter, prospective trial: Endovascular Atherectomy Safety and Effectiveness (EASE) study (NCT01541774). The EASE study enrolled 129 patients with 149 lesions, 32% of the patients had CLI with 52% tibial target lesions. Atherectomy was coupled with adjunctive PTA in 85% of the patients. The primary endpoint of technical success was greater than 95.1% — compared with a target performance goal of greater than 86%; 6-month freedom from TLR was 88%. Major adverse event rate was 5.7% with a 2.9% unplanned amputation rate, 1.9% perforation rate, and 0.9% distal embolization rate. Further experience in larger studies with both technologies in the CLI population is needed before the efficacy and safety can truly be evaluated.

Orbital atherectomy using the CSI platform has gained use both in the peripheral and coronary circulations. The purported mechanism is ablation of plaque and calcium to improve vessel compliance. The catheter has an ability to ablate plaque in a variety of vessel sizes by using 1 atherectomy crown by varying speed. The performance of orbital atherectomy for CLI has been evaluated in several clinical studies and registries.[41,42] The COMPLIANCE 360° Trial (a randomized, prospective, multicenter, pilot study comparing acute and long-term results of orbital atherectomy to balloon angioplasty for calcified femoropopliteal disease) demonstrated that orbital atherectomy coupled with PTA compared with PTA alone was associated with a numerically lower (but not statistically significant) need for bailout stenting.[34,41] Larger randomized data for this device in treatment of CLI are lacking at this time.

WHICH THERAPIES ARE BEST?

Ultimately, choosing the right devices and measures of success remains more complicated than it may seem in the context of CLI. Initial limb salvage or wound closure means little if there is aggressive target vessel failure and early symptom recurrence. The endovascular approaches highlighted previously vary in their acute ability to restore luminal patency and maintain durability. Durability has long been the domain of open surgical bypass. It is, however, unclear whether longer-term patency (1 year or more) is relevant in CLI. Despite the high recurrence rate of foot ulcers, revascularization and successful wound closure coupled with preventative therapy can be effective in reducing future limb events. Meta-analyses of studies comparing PTA/endovascular therapy with open surgery for CLI have confirmed the superior performance of surgery for patency — but have failed to demonstrate differences in limb salvage rates.[43] These findings imply that lower extremity ulcer healing is a process that is dependent on early arterial patency in the context of adequate wound care.

SUMMARY

CLI remains an important cause of significant morbidity and mortality. Although few randomized data are available, an endovascular first seems an acceptable alternative to open surgery, especially in patients with high risk of morbidity and mortality in the perioperative setting. Specific outcomes in the CLI population vary among trials related to a variety of endovascular therapies, patient populations, and inconsistent administration and reporting of adjunctive wound care. Newer therapeutic options for endovascular therapies, such as atherectomy devices and DCBs, may improve procedural outcomes and durability but remain to be rigorously studied in the CLI population.

REFERENCES

1. Fowkes FG, Rudan D, Rudan I, et al. Comparison of global estimates of prevalence and risk factors for peripheral artery disease in 2000 and 2010: a systematic review and analysis. Lancet 2013;382:1329–40.
2. Reinecke H, Unrath M, Freisinger E, et al. Peripheral arterial disease and critical limb ischaemia: still poor outcomes and lack of guideline adherence. Eur Heart J 2015;36:932–8.
3. Fortington LV, Geertzen JH, van Netten JJ, et al. Short and long term mortality rates after a lower limb amputation. Eur J Vasc Endovasc Surg 2013; 46:124–31.
4. Lambert MA, Belch JJ. Medical management of critical limb ischaemia: where do we stand today? J Intern Med 2013;274:295–307.
5. Agarwal S, Sud K, Shishehbor MH. Nationwide trends of hospital admission and outcomes among critical limb ischemia patients: from 2003-2011. J Am Coll Cardiol 2016;67:1901–13.
6. Gerhard-Herman MD, Gornik HL, Barrett C, et al. 2016 AHA/ACC guideline on the management of

patients with lower extremity peripheral artery disease: a report of the American College of Cardiology/American Heart Association Task Force on Clinical Practice Guidelines. J Am Coll Cardiol 2016. [Epub ahead of print].

7. Antithrombotic Trialists Collaboration. Collaborative meta-analysis of randomised trials of antiplatelet therapy for prevention of death, myocardial infarction, and stroke in high risk patients. BMJ 2002;324:71–86.

8. Berger JS, Krantz MJ, Kittelson JM, et al. Aspirin for the prevention of cardiovascular events in patients with peripheral artery disease: a meta-analysis of randomized trials. JAMA 2009;301:1909–19.

9. CAPRIE Steering Committee. A randomised, blinded, trial of clopidogrel versus aspirin in patients at risk of ischaemic events (CAPRIE). CAPRIE Steering Committee. Lancet 1996;348:1329–39.

10. Hiatt WR, Fowkes FGR, Heizer G et al. Ticagrelor versus clopidogrel in symptomatic peripheral artery disease. N Eng J Med.

11. Patterson C, Stouffer GA, Madamanchi N, et al. New tricks for old dogs: nonthrombotic effects of thrombin in vessel wall biology. Circ Res 2001;88:987–97.

12. Morrow DA, Braunwald E, Bonaca MP, et al. Vorapaxar in the secondary prevention of atherothrombotic events. N Engl J Med 2012;366:1404–13.

13. Bonaca MP, Scirica BM, Creager MA, et al. Vorapaxar in patients with peripheral artery disease: results from TRA2{degrees}P-TIMI 50. Circulation 2013;127:1522–9, 1529e1–6.

14. Heart Protection Study Collaborative Group. Randomized trial of the effects of cholesterol-lowering with simvastatin on peripheral vascular and other major vascular outcomes in 20,536 people with peripheral arterial disease and other high-risk conditions. J Vasc Surg 2007;45:645–54 [discussion: 653–4].

15. Kumbhani DJ, Steg PG, Cannon CP, et al. Statin therapy and long-term adverse limb outcomes in patients with peripheral artery disease: insights from the REACH registry. Eur Heart J 2014;35:2864–72.

16. Ostergren J, Sleight P, Dagenais G, et al. Impact of ramipril in patients with evidence of clinical or subclinical peripheral arterial disease. Eur Heart J 2004; 25:17–24.

17. Hoel AW, Nolan BW, Goodney PP, et al. Variation in smoking cessation after vascular operations. J Vasc Surg 2013;57:1338–44 [quiz: 1344.e1–4].

18. Armstrong EJ, Wu J, Singh GD, et al. Smoking cessation is associated with decreased mortality and improved amputation-free survival among patients with symptomatic peripheral artery disease. J Vasc Surg 2014;60:1565–71.

19. Clair C, Rigotti NA, Porneala B, et al. Association of smoking cessation and weight change with cardiovascular disease among adults with and without diabetes. JAMA 2013;309:1014–21.

20. Selvarajah S, Black JH 3rd, Malas MB, et al. Preoperative smoking is associated with early graft failure after infrainguinal bypass surgery. J Vasc Surg 2014; 59:1308–14.

21. Adam DJ, Beard JD, Cleveland T, et al. Bypass versus angioplasty in severe ischaemia of the leg (BASIL): multicentre, randomised controlled trial. Lancet 2005;366:1925–34.

22. Menard MT, Farber A, Assmann SF, et al. Design and rationale of the best endovascular versus best surgical therapy for patients with critical limb ischemia (BEST-CLI) trial. J Am Heart Assoc 2016;5(7):e003219.

23. Tepe G, Laird J, Schneider P, et al. Drug-coated balloon versus standard percutaneous transluminal angioplasty for the treatment of superficial femoral and popliteal peripheral artery disease: 12-month results from the IN.PACT SFA randomized trial. Circulation 2015;131:495–502.

24. Liistro F, Porto I, Angioli P, et al. Drug-eluting balloon in peripheral intervention for below the knee angioplasty evaluation (DEBATE-BTK): a randomized trial in diabetic patients with critical limb ischemia. Circulation 2013;128:615–21.

25. Zeller T, Baumgartner I, Scheinert D, et al. Drug-eluting balloon versus standard balloon angioplasty for infrapopliteal arterial revascularization in critical limb ischemia: 12-month results from the IN.PACT DEEP randomized trial. J Am Coll Cardiol 2014;64:1568–76.

26. Schillinger M, Sabeti S, Loewe C, et al. Balloon angioplasty versus implantation of nitinol stents in the superficial femoral artery. N Engl J Med 2006;354: 1879–88.

27. Feiring AJ, Krahn M, Nelson L, et al. Preventing leg amputations in critical limb ischemia with below-the-knee drug-eluting stents: the PaRADISE (PReventing Amputations using Drug eluting StEnts) trial. J Am Coll Cardiol 2010;55:1580–9.

28. Rocha-Singh KJ, Jaff M, Joye J, et al. Major adverse limb events and wound healing following infrapopliteal artery stent implantation in patients with critical limb ischemia: the XCELL trial. Catheter Cardiovasc Interv 2012;80:1042–51.

29. Trombert D, Caradu C, Brizzi V, et al. Evidence for the use of drug eluting stents in below-the-knee lesions. J Cardiovasc Surg (Torino) 2015;56:67–71.

30. Fusaro M, Cassese S, Ndrepepa G, et al. Drug-eluting stents for revascularization of infrapopliteal arteries: updated meta-analysis of randomized trials. JACC Cardiovasc Interv 2013;6:1284–93.

31. Varcoe RL, Schouten O, Thomas SD, et al. Experience with the absorb everolimus-eluting bioresorbable vascular scaffold in arteries below the knee: 12-Month clinical and imaging outcomes. JACC Cardiovasc Interv 2016;9:1721–8.

32. Panaich SS, Arora S, Patel N, et al. In-hospital outcomes of atherectomy during endovascular lower

extremity revascularization. Am J Cardiol 2016;117: 676–84.

33. Jones WS, Mi X, Qualls LG, et al. Trends in settings for peripheral vascular intervention and the effect of changes in the outpatient prospective payment system. J Am Coll Cardiol 2015;65:920–7.

34. Lee MS, Mustapha J, Beasley R, et al. Impact of lesion location on procedural and acute angiographic outcomes in patients with critical limb ischemia treated for peripheral artery disease with orbital atherectomy: A CONFIRM registries subanalysis. Catheter Cardiovasc Interv 2016;87: 440–5.

35. Todd KE Jr, Ahanchi SS, Maurer CA, et al. Atherectomy offers no benefits over balloon angioplasty in tibial interventions for critical limb ischemia. J Vasc Surg 2013;58:941–8.

36. Laird JR, Zeller T, Gray BH, et al. Limb salvage following laser-assisted angioplasty for critical limb ischemia: results of the LACI multicenter trial. J Endovasc Ther 2006;13:1–11.

37. McKinsey JF, Zeller T, Rocha-Singh KJ, et al. Lower extremity revascularization using directional atherectomy: 12-month prospective results of the DEFINITIVE LE study. JACC Cardiovasc Interv 2014;7:923–33.

38. Peripheral atherectomy with the Rotablator: a multicenter report. The Collaborative Rotablator Atherectomy Group (CRAG). J Vasc Surg 1994;19: 509–15.

39. Sixt S, Scheinert D, Rastan A, et al. One-year outcome after percutaneous rotational and aspiration atherectomy in infrainguinal arteries in patient with and without type 2 diabetes mellitus. Ann Vasc Surg 2011;25:520–9.

40. Sixt S, Rastan A, Scheinert D, et al. The 1-year clinical impact of rotational aspiration atherectomy of infrainguinal lesions. Angiology 2011;62:645–56.

41. Dattilo R, Himmelstein SI, Cuff RF. The COMPLIANCE 360 degrees Trial: a randomized, prospective, multicenter, pilot study comparing acute and long-term results of orbital atherectomy to balloon angioplasty for calcified femoropopliteal disease. J Invasive Cardiol 2014;26:355–60.

42. Lee MS, Yang T, Adams G. Pooled analysis of the CONFIRM registries: safety outcomes in diabetic patients treated with orbital atherectomy for peripheral artery disease. J Endovasc Ther 2014;21:258–65.

43. Romiti M, Albers M, Brochado-Neto FC, et al. Meta-analysis of infrapopliteal angioplasty for chronic critical limb ischemia. J Vasc Surg 2008; 47:975–81.

Inframalleolar Intervention for Limb Preservation

Javier A. Valle, MD, MSc[a], Andrew F. Prouse, MD[b], Robert K. Rogers, MD, MSc, RPVI[c],*

KEYWORDS

- Critical limb ischemia • Endovascular interventions • Pedal interventions
- Inframalleolar interventions • Limb salvage • Peripheral vascular disease

---

KEY POINTS

- Critical limb ischemia (CLI) portends a high risk of amputation and death. Revascularization is a mainstay of therapy for patients with CLI.
- There is a high prevalence of tibioperoneal and pedal arterial disease in patients with CLI.
- Advanced endovascular therapies are evolving to revascularize distal, small-vessel disease.
- The ability to revascularize inframalleolar arterial disease is improving due to increased operator experience and emerging technologies; however, there remains an evidence gap in this field.

INTRODUCTION

Critical limb ischemia (CLI) is defined as ischemic rest pain or tissue loss in the setting of reduced limb perfusion. CLI is a relatively prevalent condition, estimated to occur in 35 per 10,000 patients annually[1] in the United States, and is associated with significant morbidity and poor outcomes. Retrospective analyses of patients suffering from CLI have demonstrated a risk of amputation up to 67% at 4 years[2] and a 2-year mortality of nearly 40%.[3] Even in the setting of regular follow-up provided in clinical trials, patients with CLI who are unable to undergo revascularization have amputation rates of 21% and mortality rates of 15% at 1 year.[4] Given the poor prognosis these patients face, improved CLI therapies are needed.

Revascularization is a mainstay of CLI therapy. Unfortunately, many patients with CLI are considered unsuitable for revascularization. Surgical options are often limited by prohibitive

operative risk in this patient population with a high prevalence of comorbidities such as diabetes mellitus, active tobacco use, increased age, renal failure, and coronary or cerebrovascular disease.[4,5] A second challenge of surgical revascularization is the high prevalence of tibioperoneal and pedal disease in CLI, which comprises distal bypass targets. For example, in a retrospective study of 450 patients with CLI undergoing catheter-based angiography at 2 academic institutions, the prevalence of popliteal or infrapopliteal occlusions was 91%.[6] The high prevalence of diabetes mellitus in CLI populations undoubtedly contributes to this preponderance of small-vessel disease.[7]

For these reasons, endovascular therapy for CLI has gained appeal. Bolstering the enthusiasm for percutaneous strategies is the concept of "angiosomes," wherein each below-knee vessel is considered responsible for perfusing distinct areas of the lower extremity. Based on this concept, clinicians have more recently invoked

---

Dr R.K. Rogers is on the adjudication committee for VOYAGER, funded by Bayer. Dr J.A. Valle is a subinvestigator for VOYAGER, funded by Bayer.

[a] Division of Cardiology, University of Colorado School of Medicine, 12361 East 17th Avenue, Box 130, Aurora, CO 80045, USA; [b] Division of Cardiology, University of Colorado School of Medicine, University of Colorado, Mail Stop B132, Academic Office 1, Office 7104, Aurora, CO 80045, USA; [c] Vascular Medicine & Intervention, Interventional Cardiology, Division of Cardiology, University of Colorado School of Medicine, University of Colorado, Mail Stop B132, Leprino Building, 12401 East 17th Avenue, Room 560, Aurora, CO 80045, USA
* Corresponding author.
E-mail address: kevin.rogers@ucdenver.edu

Intervent Cardiol Clin 6 (2017) 261–270
http://dx.doi.org/10.1016/j.iccl.2016.12.009

an angiosome-driven approach to revascularization, specifically targeting the vessel believed to provide direct blood flow to a wound.[8,9] As such, operators increasingly perform tibioperoneal and pedal interventions with the goal of providing direct, in-line flow to the angiosome of interest, rather than only revascularizing the aorto-iliac or femoral-popliteal "inflow." This increased experience, coupled with devices designed for pedal intervention, are establishing a new paradigm for CLI therapy.

In this review, we describe an approach to pedal interventions. An overview of the assessment of foot perfusion is provided, followed by a review of devices for inframalleolar intervention, procedural considerations, and emerging techniques.

ASSESSMENT OF FOOT PERFUSION

The ability to assess pedal perfusion accurately is a major challenge in the field of CLI. Nonetheless, it is critical for the interventionalist to consider foot perfusion for multiple reasons:

- To identify patients with poor perfusion in the angiosome of interest who might benefit from revascularization.
- To identify patients with seemingly adequate perfusion who may not benefit from revascularization and who would be exposed unnecessarily to procedural risks.
- To select a target vessel for revascularization.
- To understand when revascularization is complete versus when further endovascular therapy should be pursued.

Various modalities for assessing pedal perfusion are listed in Table 1. The ideal test for pedal perfusion would be inexpensive, readily available, reproducible, and improve the clinician's ability to predict outcomes. Additionally, the ideal test would be "angiosome-specific"; that is, perfusion data could be obtained from any angiosome of interest in the foot. Currently, there are limitations of each modality for assessing pedal perfusion, and more research is needed in this field (Fig. 1).

TECHNOLOGY FOR INFRAMALLEOLAR INTERVENTION

Devices dedicated for pedal intervention are emerging (Table 2). Angioplasty balloons are now available for small-diameter arteries in the foot with sufficient shaft lengths to reach the foot from contralateral femoral access. Likewise, several atherectomy devices may increase technical success rates for pedal intervention. Specific access kits also exist for the foot. Finally, a platform for arterialization of infrapopliteal veins is being tested (Fig. 2).

PROCEDURAL CONSIDERATIONS FOR INFRAMALLEOLAR INTERVENTION

Access

When considering access, it should be recognized that most pedal lesions to be treated are occlusions, rather than stenoses, and may or may not be contiguous with supramalleolar occlusions. Choosing site(s) that allow access to the proximal and distal caps of the occlusion can increase the chance of procedural success. Although contralateral femoral access is an option for pedal revascularization, the authors rarely choose this access site because of limitations in the length of equipment and decreased catheter "pushability" compared with ipsilateral limb access. Rather, nontraditional access is often obtained.

Table 1 Modalities for assessing pedal perfusion		
Modality	**Advantages**	**Disadvantages**
Ankle-brachial index	Inexpensive Readily available Large evidence base	Noncompressibility Not consistent with angiosome hypothesis
Toe pressure	Inexpensive Readily available	Does not provide information on all parts of the foot
Transcutaneous oximetry	Provides angiosome-specific data	Large coefficient of variation
Skin perfusion pressure	Provides angiosome-specific data	Limited evidence base Little correlation with outcomes
Two-dimensional perfusion imaging	Provides intraprocedural, angiosome-specific data	Emerging technology with limited evidence base and no correlation with outcomes

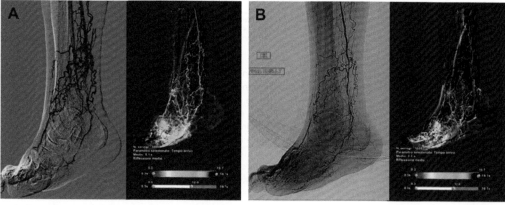

Fig. 1. Two-dimensional (2D) perfusion imaging. Parameters of contrast delivery to the foot are quantified to generate a color map of pedal perfusion. (A) Before revascularization of the posterior tibial artery. (B) Post revascularization angiogram and 2D perfusion image.

Antegrade common femoral artery access

This site is a mainstay for pedal intervention. Our default strategy is to use this site to access the proximal cap of tibioperoneal and pedal occlusions. This access site allows in-line "pushability," which facilitates successful crossing of occlusions and provides adequate proximity to the ipsilateral foot such that equipment length is rarely an issue. The common femoral artery also can accommodate practically any size of device that might be needed for pedal intervention. The antegrade common femoral artery access site is typically used to deliver therapy, although dedicated pedal technology also permits treating distal disease from the foot. At times, body habitus can make antegrade femoral access challenging. Hemostasis is at the discretion of the operator. For most pedal interventions, a small-bore sheath is sufficient (5F), and as such we prefer manual compression, although closure devices are an option.

Tibioperoneal access

Retrograde tibioperoneal access is often used to treat tibioperoneal occlusions. This access site, however, clearly orients the operator away from the foot and, therefore, is rarely useful in pedal intervention. Antegrade tibioperoneal

Table 2			
Examples of devices for inframalleolar intervention			
Device	**Company**	**Use**	**Vessel Size**
170-mm shaft angioplasty balloon	Cook (Bloomington, Indiana)	Pedal intervention from contralateral femoral access	2.5 mm
1.25-mm Micro-crown	CSI (St. Paul, MN)	Orbital atherectomy	1.5 mm
0.9-mm laser catheter	Spectranetics (Colorado Springs, CO)	Photoablation	2.0 mm
DS Silverhawk catheter	Medtronic (Minneapolis, MN)	Excisional atherectomy	1.5 mm
Micropuncture kit	Cook (Bloomington, Indiana)	Pedal access allowing 2.6F catheter through 2.9F sheath	~1.5 mm
LimFlow device • 7F arterial "send" catheter • 5F venous "receive" catheter	MD Start (Paris, France)	Percutaneous deep vein arterialization of infrapopliteal veins, via ultrasonographic positioning of arterial and venous catheters and formation of arteriovenous fistula for crossover and arterialization of the deep veins	Results in increased perfusion of all vessel sizes

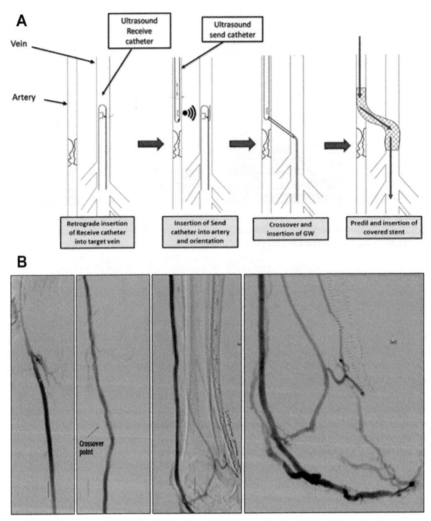

Fig. 2. Percutaneous venous arterialization of the foot. (A) Schematic of technique for percutaneous venous arterialization. (B) Final angiogram following procedure.

access is an option to provide access to the distal cap of a pedal artery occlusion.

Alternative access to the distal cap of an inframalleolar occlusion

Pedal-plantar loop approach. The plantar arch (anastomosis of the dorsalis pedis and lateral plantar arteries) can be used to gain access to the distal cap of inframalleolar occlusions (Fig. 3). The "deep arch" of the foot connects the medial plantar artery with the lateral tarsal branch, and can be navigated in a similar fashion to the plantar arch. Care must be taken to avoid spasm and unnecessary trauma to this delicate vasculature.

Transcollateral approach. Collaterals also can provide access to the distal cap of below-knee occlusions (Fig. 4).[10] In particular, 2 naturally occurring anastomoses occur at the ankle: the anterior communicating artery connects the anterior tibial and peroneal arteries, and the posterior communicating artery connects the posterior tibial and peroneal arteries. These pathways are more useful for tibioperoneal, rather than pedal, interventions, however.

Metatarsal access
Transmetatarsal access has been described (Fig. 5).[11] In a series of 28 patients with CLI, Palena and Manzi[11] described obtaining transmetatarsal access of the 1st dorsal artery (n = 25) and plantar arch (n = 3) to facilitate pedal and tibioperoneal revascularization, achieving a procedural success rate of 88%.

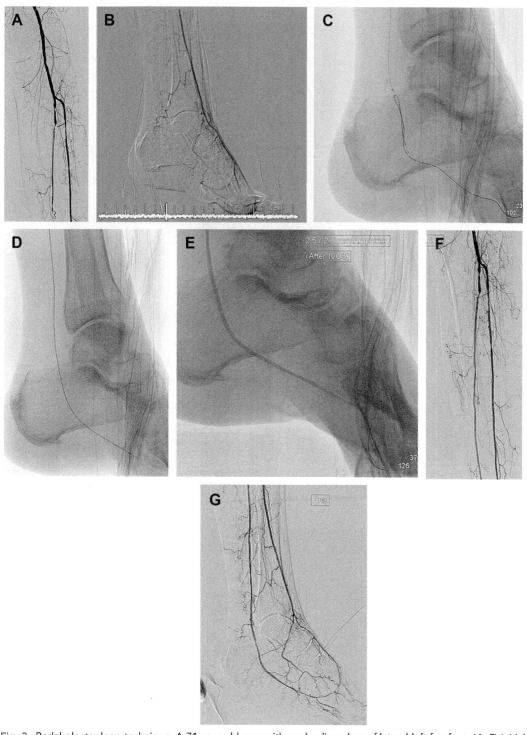

Fig. 3. Pedal-plantar loop technique. A 71-year-old man with nonhealing ulcer of lateral left forefoot. (*A, B*) Initial angiogram taken from antegrade ipsilateral femoral sheath with tip in popliteal artery. Note posterior tibial artery occlusion contiguous with lateral plantar occlusion in the foot. (*C*) Wire advanced retrograde across lateral plantar (pedal-plantar loop technique) to facilitate antegrade crossing. (*D*) Orbital atherectomy of posterior tibial and lateral plantar arteries. (*E*) Intravascular ultrasound (IVUS)-guided angioplasty of posterior tibial and lateral plantar arteries. (*F, G*) Final angiography showing revascularized posterior tibial and lateral plantar arteries.

A

B

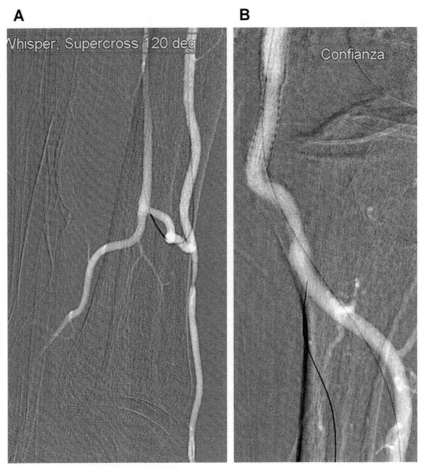

Fig. 4. Transcollateral access to facilitate retrograde crossing of peroneal occlusion. (A) Anterior communicating artery is traversed from anterior tibial into peroneal artery. (B) Retrograde crossing of peroneal occlusion.

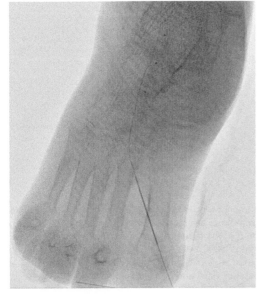

Fig. 5. Transmetatarsal access.

Antithrombotic Therapy

There are no data as of yet to guide the use of specific antithrombotic therapy for pedal intervention. In the absence of evidence, the authors prefer to use unfractionated heparin with a goal activated clotting time of 300 to 350 seconds during inframalleolar procedures. We also favor at least aspirin for antiplatelet therapy intraprocedurally. Postprocedurally, we prescribe dual antiplatelet therapy until wound healing occurs. Dual antiplatelet therapy typically includes aspirin 81 mg daily but the preferable second agent is under investigation.[12,13] Anticoagulation in addition to aspirin versus aspirin alone in patients who have undergone an endovascular procedure for symptomatic peripheral arterial disease is also being investigated.[14] Upcoming trials in populations with peripheral arterial disease are encouraging. However, the evidence generated for antithrombotic therapy that is specifically generalizable to inframalleolar disease may be sparse.

Crossing

Crossing inframalleolar occlusions is often the most challenging step of the procedure. Our default strategy is to cross antegrade if the anatomy appears unambiguous (Fig. 6). There are number of available 0.014-inch and 0.018-inch wires and support catheters dedicated to crossing infrapopliteal occlusions. If true lumen crossing is achieved, then the crossing wire can be exchanged for a working wire and therapy delivered. It is not uncommon, however, that crossing is achieved in a subintimal plane, particularly if the inframalleolar occlusion is contiguous with a long tibial occlusion. In the absence of dedicated reentry devices for the foot, we favor resolving the subintimal space by crossing retrograde. If the retrograde wire crosses true lumen, then the retrograde wire can be externalized, reversed, and then therapy delivered. If the retrograde wire is also subintimal, then techniques such as CART (controlled antegrade and retrograde tracking) or SAFARI (subintimal arterial flossing with antegrade-retrograde

intervention) can be used, whereby subintimal angioplasty is performed to join the antegrade and retrograde subintimal spaces to allow true lumen reentry.[15]

Therapy

There are no randomized trials comparing available therapies for inframalleolar interventions; however, there is observational evidence that pedal interventions can be performed successfully and safely. A total of 135 patients underwent revascularization of the pedal vasculature by using the pedal-plantar loop technique, with an acute success (as defined by the ability to perform balloon angioplasty with adequate angiographic result) in 85%.[16] Angioplasty is a cornerstone of therapy. We promote the use of intravascular ultrasound to properly size the vessel, which maximizes the chance of acute lumen gain without dissection (Fig. 7). There is little or no evidence on reports of pedal atherectomy. The smallest orbital atherectomy catheter is designed to treat

A

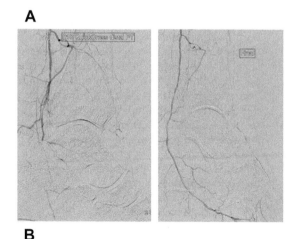

B

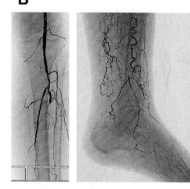
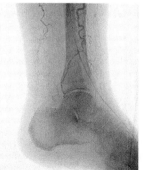
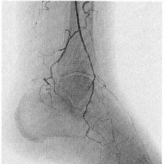

Fig. 6. Crossing of long-segment occlusions. (A) Example of unambiguous proximal cap that facilitated antegrade true lumen crossing of the lateral plantar artery. (B) Example of ambiguous proximal cap of apparent anterior tibial artery occlusion in patient with first toe wound. Due to ambiguous proximal cap, the dorsalis pedis was accessed for retrograde crossing. After revascularization, it became apparent that the peroneal artery supplied the dorsalis pedis, a congenital variant.

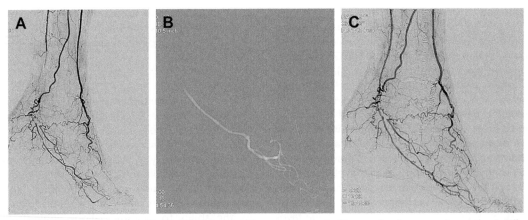

Fig. 7. Plantar artery revascularization. An 88-year-old man presented with a nonhealing wound over the Achilles tendon. (A) Initial angiography. (B) Selective lateral plantar fluoroscopic roadmap to confirm true lumen position following antegrade crossing. (C) Final angiography following orbital atherectomy and IVUS-guided angioplasty with nitinol-caged and scoring balloons.

vessels as small as 1.5 mm. Because of the high prevalence of calcification in below-knee arteries in patients with critical limb ischemia, orbital atherectomy can be a useful adjunct to angioplasty for pedal intervention, but should be used with care (Fig. 8), as safety data for this specific anatomic subset is not yet available. Excisional atherectomy catheters have been designed for vessels as small as 1.5 mm, as well. Similarly, laser ablation catheters have been designed to treat vessels as small as 2.0 mm, but there is lack of data on the use of this technology specifically for pedal revascularization. Stenting of the dorsalis pedis has been reported.[17,18] In a case series of 11 patients treated with balloon-expandable

drug-eluting stents deployed below the ankle, restenosis rates were 50% at 6 months. Stent compression, fracture, or deformation developed in 5 (45%) of 11 patients, with 1 case resulting in recurrent CLI and major amputation.[18] In another series of 8 patients undergoing bare metal stenting in the dorsalis pedis for limb salvage, acute or subacute thrombosis developed in 25% (n = 2) and restenosis occurred in 50% (n = 4). Of the 8 patients in this series undergoing stenting, 7 demonstrated complete wound healing. However, stent deformity or fracture occurred in 87.5% of patients (n = 7).[17] It is the authors' opinion that stenting of inframalleolar vessels should be avoided, if possible.

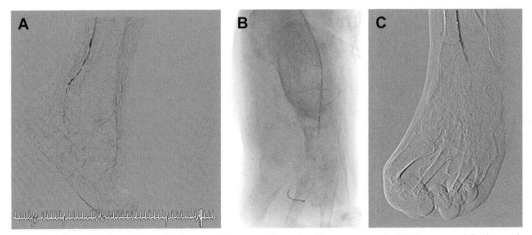

Fig. 8. Pedal artery atherectomy. An 88-year-old man with nonhealing toe wounds. (A) Severe pedal atherosclerotic disease. (B) Orbital atherectomy of dorsalis pedis. (C) "No reflow" following atherectomy.

SUMMARY

Endovascular therapy for inframalleolar disease is an important part of the multiple facets of care that are essential for optimal outcomes in patients with CLI; that is, pedal revascularization should be performed in concert with meticulous wound care, treatment of infection, control of diabetes, optimizing nutrition, and often foot surgery. Nonetheless, the ability of operators to now revascularize the foot is expected to improve outcomes in patients with CLI, but this notion is yet to be proven.

Although the progress made in revascularization of distal disease for CLI is exciting and encouraging, there remains work to be done in this field. Improvements in the ability to assess pedal perfusion are needed. Additionally, integrating the assessment of foot perfusion into clinical decision-making and prognostication is necessary. Due to the complex technical nature of pedal intervention and the resources necessary to provide complete care for the patient with CLI, CLI Centers of Excellence are needed so that all patients with CLI have access to optimal revascularization options and comprehensive CLI care. The technical advances to date are promising, as are therapeutic options on the horizon, such as arterialization of below-knee veins. However, future devices are needed, such as dedicated pedal stents, drug-eluting devices for the foot, and access to equipment designed for metatarsal arteries.

Finally, like most areas in CLI, there is a profound evidence gap in inframalleolar intervention. Observational studies with safety and efficacy data focused on pedal intervention are needed. Fortunately, the recently completed observational study, of LIBERTY, is anticipated to contribute relevant data.[19,20] The clinical utility of pedal revascularization should be investigated. Eventually, randomized trials of pedal interventional techniques and devices should be performed.

In conclusion, inframalleolar intervention provides another tool in the armamentarium of the total care of the patient with CLI and provides another step forward in the treatment of this challenging disease.

REFERENCES

1. Nehler MR, Duval S, Diao L, et al. Epidemiology of peripheral arterial disease and critical limb ischemia in an insured national population. J Vasc Surg 2014;60:686–95.e2.

2. Reinecke H, Unrath M, Freisinger E, et al. Peripheral arterial disease and critical limb ischaemia: still poor outcomes and lack of guideline adherence. Eur Heart J 2015;36:932–8.

3. Soga Y, Iida O, Takahara M, et al. Two-year life expectancy in patients with critical limb ischemia. JACC Cardiovasc Interv 2014;7:1444–9.

4. Belch J, Hiatt WR, Baumgartner I, et al. Effect of fibroblast growth factor NV1FGF on amputation and death: a randomised placebo-controlled trial of gene therapy in critical limb ischaemia. Lancet 2011;377:1929–37.

5. Adam DJ, Beard JD, Cleveland T, et al. Bypass versus angioplasty in severe ischaemia of the leg (BASIL): multicentre, randomised controlled trial. Lancet 2005;366:1925–34.

6. Rueda CA, Nehler MR, Perry DJ, et al. Patterns of artery disease in 450 patients undergoing revascularization for critical limb ischemia: implications for clinical trial design. J Vasc Surg 2008;47:995–9 [discussion: 999–1000].

7. Ciavarella A, Silletti A, Mustacchio A, et al. Angiographic evaluation of the anatomic pattern of arterial obstructions in diabetic patients with critical limb ischaemia. Diabete Metab 1993;19:586–9.

8. McCallum JC, Lane JS. 3rd. Angiosome-directed revascularization for critical limb ischemia. Semin Vasc Surg 2014;27:32–7.

9. Dieter RS, Dieter RA, Dieter RA, SpringerLink. Endovascular interventions: a case-based approach. New York: Springer; 2014.

10. Fusaro M, Agostoni P, Biondi-Zoccai G. "Transcollateral" angioplasty for a challenging chronic total occlusion of the tibial vessels: a novel approach to percutaneous revascularization in critical lower limb ischemia. Catheter Cardiovasc Interv 2008; 71:268–72.

11. Palena LM, Manzi M. Extreme below-the-knee interventions: retrograde transmetatarsal or transplantar arch access for foot salvage in challenging cases of critical limb ischemia. J Endovasc Ther 2012;19:805–11.

12. Berger JS, Katona BG, Jones WS, et al. Design and rationale for the Effects of Ticagrelor and Clopidogrel in Patients with Peripheral Artery Disease (EUCLID) trial. Am Heart J 2016;175: 86–93.

13. Bhatt DL, Flather MD, Hacke W, et al. Patients with prior myocardial infarction, stroke, or symptomatic peripheral arterial disease in the CHARISMA trial. J Am Coll Cardiol 2007;49:1982–8.

14. Efficacy and safety of rivaroxaban in reducing the risk of major thrombotic vascular events in subjects with symptomatic peripheral artery disease undergoing peripheral revascularization procedures of the lower extremities (VOYAGER PAD). 2016.

15. Rogers RK, Dattilo PB, Garcia JA, et al. Retrograde approach to recanalization of complex tibial disease. Catheter Cardiovasc Interv 2011;77:915–25.

16. Manzi M, Fusaro M, Ceccacci T, et al. Clinical results of below-the knee intervention using pedal-plantar loop technique for the revascularization of foot arteries. J Cardiovasc Surg 2009;50:331–7.

17. Kawarada O, Yokoi Y, Higashimori A, et al. Stent-assisted below-the-ankle angioplasty for limb salvage. J Endovasc Ther 2011;18:32–42.

18. Katsanos K, Diamantopoulos A, Spiliopoulos S, et al. Below-the-ankle angioplasty and stenting for limb salvage: anatomical considerations and long-term outcomes. Cardiovasc Intervent Radiol 2013;36:926–35.

19. Adams GL, Mustapha J, Gray W, et al. The LIBERTY study: design of a prospective, observational, multicenter trial to evaluate the acute and long-term clinical and economic outcomes of real-world endovascular device interventions in treating peripheral artery disease. Am Heart J 2016;174:14–21.

20. Observational study to evaluate PAD treatment clinical and economic outcomes (LIBERTY). 2013.

Angiosome-Guided Intervention in Critical Limb Ischemia

Matthew C. Bunte, MD, MS[a],*,
Mehdi H. Shishehbor, DO, MPH, PhD[b]

KEYWORDS

• Critical limb ischemia • Angiosome • Revascularization • Limb reperfusion

---

KEY POINTS

- Successful revascularization for CLI involves knowledge of limb perfusion strategy, technical expertise in reperfusion therapies, and an approach of multidisciplinary care to address complex patient comorbidities.
- Broad conclusions about CLI reperfusion strategy are challenged by the heterogeneous and generally nonrandomized nature of available clinical studies.
- Although these observational analyses have limitations, they provide contemporary evidence of real-world limb revascularization that substantiate further clinical use and study of angiosome-directed limb reperfusion.

INTRODUCTION

Although accounting for a minority 1% to 3% of the more than 8 million Americans affected by peripheral artery disease (PAD), critical limb ischemia (CLI) is associated with substantial risks of limb loss, health care resource utilization, and high rates of fatal vascular and nonvascular events.[1–3] CLI represents the terminal consequences of severe PAD, including chronic ischemic rest pain, arterial ulceration, and gangrene. Revascularization is the optimal treatment of CLI to relieve ischemic limb pain, promote limb salvage, and to avoid major amputation.[2]

Effective arterial reperfusion is marked by improved hemodynamics to the distal extremity and at the wound bed. Evidence supports the use of either bypass surgery or endovascular therapy to that end.[4] Advances in technology that facilitate arterial revascularization, particularly endovascular techniques, have expanded treatment options for those with complex PAD and have been expertly reviewed elsewhere.[5] Several key factors should be considered in selecting a revascularization strategy, including the patient's operative risk, location of ischemia, and anatomic pattern of arterial disease. Evolution of limb reperfusion strategy also helps to shape how revascularization is applied to maximize opportunity for wound healing and limb salvage.

In recent years, angiosome-directed revascularization has developed into a popular theory of reperfusion, whereby anatomically directed arterial flow is restored to the wound bed. Clinical evidence continues to mount as to the efficacy of this strategy, although important limitations remain. This state-of-the-art review evaluates the development of the angiosome-directed model of revascularization for CLI, explores the current evidence supporting its use especially for infrapopliteal arterial revascularization, and

---

Grant Support: None.
Relationships: None.
a Saint Luke's Mid America Heart Institute, St Luke's Hospital, University of Missouri-Kansas City School of Medicine, 4401 Wornall Road, Kansas City, MO 64111, USA; b Robert and Suzanne Tomsich Department of Cardiovascular Medicine, Cleveland Clinic, 9500 Euclid Avenue, Cleveland, OH 44195, USA
* Corresponding author.
E-mail address: mbunte@saint-lukes.org

considers future implications of the angiosome model that may guide endovascular reperfusion strategies.

THE ANGIOSOME MODEL

Achieving direct, in-line arterial flow to an area of ischemic tissue is the foundation of the angiosome approach. First described within the scope of reconstructive plastic surgery, the angiosome represents a territory of vascular cascade that corresponds to a specific three-dimensional dermal topography.[6] The foot and ankle have six distinct angiosomes supplied by the three major infrapopliteal arteries (Fig. 1).[7] The posterior tibial artery contributes to three angiosomes: the medial and lateral plantar surface of the foot, and the medial surface of the heel. The peroneal artery provides flow to the lateral forefoot, ankle, and heel. The anterior tibial artery provides supply to the dorsum of the forefoot, ankle, and leg. A watershed network of collateral arteries provides anastomotic connections between adjacent angiosomes. This system

of collaterals allows tissue from a well-perfused angiosome to provide indirect flow via collaterals to an adjacent malperfused territory. Whereas the optimal revascularization result includes direct flow to the wound bed, indirect flow fed by collaterals of an adjacent angiosome may facilitate wound healing. The angiosome approach ensures that maximal arterial supply is directed to an affected region of ischemia, rather than simply improving global, nondirected limb flow.

REVASCULARIZATION STRATEGY IN THE GUIDELINES

The Inter-Society Consensus for the Management of Peripheral Arterial Disease (TASC II) guidelines for CLI give preference to endovascular revascularization over surgery when equivalent short- and long-term clinical outcomes are anticipated, although they are further refined based on the severity classification of inflow lesions.[2] Guideline updates in 2011 from the American Heart Association/American College

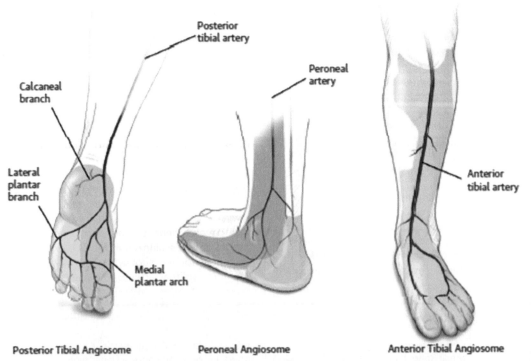

Posterior tibial artery

Peroneal artery

Calcaneal branch

Lateral plantar branch

Anterior tibial artery

Medial plantar arch

Posterior Tibial Angiosome   Peroneal Angiosome   Anterior Tibial Angiosome

Fig. 1. The below-the-knee skin and tissue are supplied by three main arteries and six angiosomes. The anterior tibial artery supplies the anterior shin and dorsum of the foot, the posterior tibial artery supplies the medial heal and the medial and lateral plantar angiosomes, and the peroneal artery supplies the lateral aspect of the heel and the lateral border of the foot. (*From* Shishehbor MH, White CJ, Gray BH, et al. Critical limb ischemia: an expert statement. J Am Coll Cardiol 2016;68:2002–15; with permission.)

of Cardiology Foundation were based on the results of BASIL, offering Class IIa recommendations that favor autologous vein grafting over balloon angioplasty when life expectancy is greater than 2 years.[8]

Although these guidelines are conceptually important, selecting a revascularization strategy requires additional consideration of patient comorbidities, variation in arterial anatomy, collateralization, prior arterial interventions, and local expertise. Assessment of distal vessel runoff relative to regional tissue ischemia and wound location is a central principle in CLI-related lower extremity revascularization. For surgical bypass, the choice of target artery is determined by factors that include surgical risk, availability of venous conduit, site of distal anastomosis, and quality of distal runoff. Endovascular techniques require consideration for feasibility to reach the target vascular bed. Often, the major arterial supply to CLI-related wounds is occluded, whereby flow to the ischemic region is delivered via a complex network of collateral vessels. In such cases, indirect revascularization with bypass grafting to improve flow into these collateral channels has been traditionally considered adequate given challenges of direct, in-line reperfusion. However, bypass graft patency alone does not ensure clinical improvement. A report from the Vascular Study Group of Northern New England registry found that 10% of patients with a patent bypass graft required major amputation or had ongoing limb ischemia 1 year after surgery.[9] In a meta-analysis of lower extremity angioplasty versus popliteal-to-distal bypass grafting, 3-year arterial patency rates were lower for angioplasty (49%) than bypass surgery (72%), although limb salvage rates were equivalent at 82%.[10] Regardless of modality, successful treatment of CLI requires careful consideration of anatomy before revascularization.

PRACTICAL USE OF ANGIOSOME-DIRECTED REVASCULARIZATION

The angiosome model has been developed from injecting and studying the anatomy of cadaveric specimens.[6,7] The main limitation of this model is its inability to incorporate the dynamic features of distal limb perfusion in the living subject. Therefore, several clinical studies evaluating the utility of the angiosome model have been performed to test the hypothesis that providing direct, in-line flow to the wound bed might provide the most favorable results.

Overall, rates of technical success and limb salvage using the angiosome approach are favorable. In a cross-sectional analysis, Alexandrescu and colleagues[11] studied 232 wounds among 208 patients with diabetes that underwent below-knee angioplasty. Patients were stratified before and after 2005, when a protocol for angiosome-oriented revascularization was initiated. Technical success was achieved in 79% of those treated with an angiosome-directed approach. Rates of survival were similar between groups, although freedom from amputation through 36 months was better among those treated with angiosome-directed revascularization.

Similar findings were confirmed in a registry analysis of 200 directly (54%) and 169 indirectly revascularized (46%) limbs for isolated infrapopliteal CLI using endovascular techniques.[12] Among 329 consecutive patients with Rutherford Class V (73%) and Class VI (27%) PAD and up to 4 years of follow-up, the analysis compared outcomes of amputation-free survival (AFS), major adverse limb events, and major amputation. Results were reported as unadjusted and adjusted within a 1:1 propensity analysis (n = 236 patients; 118 per group), although in either case outcomes favored a direct approach. After propensity adjustment, 4-year rates for AFS (49% vs 29%; $P = .002$), freedom from major adverse limb events (51% vs 28%; $P = .008$), and freedom from major amputation (82% vs 68%; $P = .01$) favored direct versus indirect revascularization. Overall, the rate of repeat intervention remained low at 30% and the AFS benefit for the direct group was consistent throughout follow-up.

The results of angiosome-directed reperfusion using surgical bypass have been mixed. In a review of surgical bypass of 52 nonhealing wounds over a 2-year period, Neville and colleagues[13] found that 91% of wounds healed with direct revascularization versus only 38% revascularized indirectly. Another study of 249 wounds among 228 patients with CLI who underwent surgical bypass grafting found slower healing rates among those indirectly revascularized, although rates of limb salvage were similar.[14] In this cohort, patients with end-stage renal disease seemed to especially benefit from angiosome-directed revascularization. After propensity score analysis, the rates of wound healing and limb salvage were similar between groups.

WOUND HEALING AND TISSUE HEMODYNAMICS

Regional tissue perfusion is perhaps the single most important objective provided with quality revascularization that promotes wound healing. Patients that fail to heal their wounds suffer high mortality rates. Varela and colleagues[15] found that, among patients with infrapopliteal CLI, angiosome-directed revascularization tended toward shorter healing time (71 vs 91 days; $P = .18$) and improved healing rate at 12 months (92% vs 73%; $P = .008$). In that study, patients with pedal wounds that could not be directly revascularized although had intact collaterals of the pedal arch fared better than those indirectly revascularized without pedal collaterals, with a 12-month healing rate of 85% versus 73%.

A preserved, or partially preserved, pedal arch may play an important role as the terminal cascade of perfusion to the forefoot that also influences the outcomes after CLI revascularization. In a British cohort, 167 lower extremity bypass procedures were performed among 154 patients. Patients that were revascularized with a complete or incomplete pedal arch had more complete and faster wound healing than those revascularized with no pedal arch.[16] Rates of AFS at 4 years were greatest when the pedal arch was complete (67.2%) or even incomplete (69.7%) versus when the arch was absent (45.9%), although these results were not statistically significant ($P = .388$).

When multiple vascular segments are affected, more complete, multilevel interventions may be favorable. Compared with isolated tibial artery intervention, Fernandez and colleagues[17] found that more complete, multilevel interventions of the femoropopliteal and tibial segments were associated with higher rates of healing (87% vs 69%; $P = .05$) and shorter healing times (7.7 vs 11.5 months; $P = .03$). For wounds of the distal extremity, providing complete revascularization to tibial and pedal vessels shortens time to wound healing and increases clinical success.

ANGIOSOMAL REVASCULARIZATION OF THE WOUND BED

Skin perfusion pressure (SPP) has been used to assess severity of ischemia[18] and prognosis for ulcer healing.[19] SPP is defined as the minimal external pressure at which tissue blood flow ceases,[18] and may be performed with one of three techniques: (1) radioisotope clearance, (2) photoplethysmography, or (3) laser Doppler. Among 177 patients with CLI undergoing endovascular revascularization, SPP at baseline (33 ± 22 mm Hg) roughly doubled after revascularization (57 ± 26 mm Hg).[20] Interestingly, there was a proportionately greater improvement

noted for angiosome-directed (67 ± 25 mm Hg) relative to indirect (41 ± 20 mm Hg) revascularization ($P = .0002$).[20] Wound blush after successful revascularization is associated with greater SPP, and both indicate higher rates of limb salvage.[21] In another analysis, when SPP was greater than 40 mm Hg and toe systolic pressure was greater than 30 mm Hg, there was a strong correlation with wound healing ($r = 0.69$; $P<.001$).[22] Although supportive in forecasting wound healing, SPP has not yet been shown to be predictive of major amputation.[12]

Other forms of microperfusion assessment have not found a benefit of angiosome-directed revascularization. Rother and colleagues[23] evaluated prerevascularization and postrevascularization assessment of microperfusion using white-light tissue spectrophotometry. After revascularization of 28 patients with CLI, including 17 patients receiving bypass and 11 receiving endovascular treatment, parameters of microcirculation, such as oxygen saturation, blood flow, and blood velocity, were not significantly different based on a strategy of direct and indirect revascularization of the affected angiosome.

SUMMARIZING THE EVIDENCE FOR ANGIOSOME-DIRECTED REPERFUSION

Table 1 summarizes the published studies evaluating angiosome-directed revascularization reported to date. Several of these studies have been previously featured. Efforts to summarize the outcomes associated with angiosome-directed treatment of CLI have offered mixed results, mostly because of limitations of component substudies, including a commonly retrospective study design, lack of treatment strategy, and heterogeneous definitions of study outcomes. Four major systematic reviews of angiosome-directed reperfusion have been published.[24–27] Interestingly, none of the four reviews feature the same criteria for substudy selection; therefore, each of these reviews share a common but unique cohort of studies. Three of these reviews also provide meta-analysis and summary hazard ratios for commonly reported end points, including rates of wound healing, limb salvage, and mortality.[24–26]

Wound healing and limb salvage were superior with an angiosome-directed revascularization in the three meta-analyses.[24–26] In the Sumpio analysis, the authors found that five of eight studies that reported wound healing rates found a benefit to direct revascularization, although the length of follow-up varied

Table 1
Studies evaluating the outcomes of angiosome-direct revascularization

Primary Author, Publication Year	Study Design	Limbs (Patients), n	Treatment Modality	Study Outcomes
Alexandrescu et al,[28] 2008	Retrospective	124 (98)	Endovascular	Wound healing
Neville et al,[13] 2009	Retrospective	52 (48)	Bypass surgery	Wound healing, limb salvage, mortality
Varela et al,[15] 2010	Retrospective	76 (70)	Bypass surgery and endovascular	Wound healing, limb salvage, mortality
Iida et al,[20] 2010	Retrospective	203 (177)	Endovascular	Limb salvage
Deguchi et al,[29] 2010	Retrospective	66 (61)	Bypass surgery	Wound healing, limb salvage
Alexandrescu et al,[11] 2011	Retrospective	232 (208)	Endovascular	Wound healing, limb salvage, mortality
Blanes Orti et al,[30] 2011	Retrospective	34 (32)	Endovascular	Wound healing
Azuma et al,[14] 2012	Retrospective	218 (228)	Bypass surgery	Wound healing, limb salvage
Iida et al,[12] 2012	Retrospective	369 (329)	Endovascular	Limb salvage, mortality
Soderstrom et al,[31] 2013	Retrospective	250 (226)	Endovascular	Wound healing
Kabra et al,[32] 2013	Prospective	64 (64)	Bypass surgery and endovascular	Wound healing, limb salvage, mortality
Fossaceca et al,[33] 2013	Retrospective	201 (201)	Endovascular	Wound healing, limb salvage
Rashid et al,[16] 2013	Retrospective	167 (154)	Bypass surgery	Wound healing, limb salvage
Lejay et al,[34] 2014	Retrospective	58 (54)	Bypass surgery	Limb salvage, mortality
Acin et al,[35] 2014	Retrospective	101 (92)	Endovascular	Wound healing, limb salvage, mortality
Kret et al,[36] 2014	Retrospective	97 (106)	Bypass surgery	Wound healing, limb salvage, mortality
Spillerova et al,[37] 2015	Retrospective	744 (744)	Bypass surgery and endovascular	Wound healing, limb salvage

considerably between studies.[27] Rates of limb salvage were similarly improved in the direct revascularization groups in 5 of 10 studies.[27]

SUMMARY

CLI revascularization is a complex clinical problem with significant variability among patients, reperfusion techniques, and institutional protocols for CLI management. Broad conclusions about CLI reperfusion strategy are challenged by the heterogeneous and generally nonrandomized nature of available clinical studies. Although these observational analyses have limitations, they provide contemporary evidence of real-world limb revascularization that substantiate further clinical use and study of angiosome-directed limb reperfusion.

REFERENCES

1. Hirsch AT, Haskal ZJ, Hertzer NR, et al. ACC/AHA 2005 guidelines for the management of patients with peripheral arterial disease (lower extremity, renal, mesenteric, and abdominal aortic): executive summary a collaborative report from the American Association for Vascular Surgery/Society for Vascular Surgery, Society for Cardiovascular Angiography and Interventions, Society for Vascular Medicine and Biology, Society of Interventional Radiology, and the ACC/AHA Task Force on Practice Guidelines (Writing Committee to Develop Guidelines for the Management of Patients With Peripheral Arterial Disease) endorsed by the American Association of Cardiovascular and Pulmonary Rehabilitation; National Heart, Lung, and Blood Institute; Society for Vascular Nursing; Trans-Atlantic Inter-Society Consensus; and Vascular Disease Foundation. J Am Coll Cardiol 2006;47(6):1239–312.

2. Norgren L, Hiatt WR, Dormandy JA, et al. Inter-Society Consensus for the Management of Peripheral Arterial Disease (TASC II). J Vasc Surg 2007;45(Suppl S):S5–67.

3. Mozaffarian D, Benjamin EJ, Go AS, et al. Heart disease and stroke statistics-2016 update: a report from the American Heart Association. Circulation 2016;133(4):e38–360.

4. Adam DJ, Beard JD, Cleveland T, et al. Bypass versus angioplasty in severe ischaemia of the leg (BASIL): multicentre, randomised controlled trial. Lancet 2005;366(9501):1925–34.

5. Shishehbor MH, White CJ, Gray BH, et al. Critical limb ischemia: an expert statement. J Am Coll Cardiol 2016;68(18):2002–15.

6. Taylor GI, Palmer JH. The vascular territories (angiosomes) of the body: experimental study and clinical applications. Br J Plast Surg 1987;40(2):113–41.

7. Attinger CE, Evans KK, Bulan E, et al. Angiosomes of the foot and ankle and clinical implications for limb salvage: reconstruction, incisions, and revascularization. Plast Reconstr Surg 2006;117(Suppl 7):261S–93S.

8. Rooke TW, Hirsch AT, Misra S, et al. 2011 ACCF/AHA Focused Update of the Guideline for the Management of Patients With Peripheral Artery Disease (updating the 2005 guideline): a report of the American College of Cardiology Foundation/American Heart Association Task Force on Practice Guidelines. J Am Coll Cardiol 2011;58(19):2020–45.

9. Simons JP, Goodney PP, Nolan BW, et al. Failure to achieve clinical improvement despite graft patency in patients undergoing infrainguinal lower extremity bypass for critical limb ischemia. J Vasc Surg 2010;51(6):1419–24.

10. Romiti M, Albers M, Brochado-Neto FC, et al. Meta-analysis of infrapopliteal angioplasty for chronic critical limb ischemia. J Vasc Surg 2008;47(5):975–81.

11. Alexandrescu V, Vincent G, Azdad K, et al. A reliable approach to diabetic neuroischemic foot wounds: below-the-knee angiosome-oriented angioplasty. J Endovasc Ther 2011;18(3):376–87.

12. Iida O, Soga Y, Hirano K, et al. Long-term results of direct and indirect endovascular revascularization based on the angiosome concept in patients with critical limb ischemia presenting with isolated below-the-knee lesions. J Vasc Surg 2012;55(2):363–70.e5.

13. Neville RF, Attinger CE, Bulan EJ, et al. Revascularization of a specific angiosome for limb salvage: does the target artery matter? Ann Vasc Surg 2009;23(3):367–73.

14. Azuma N, Uchida H, Kokubo T, et al. Factors influencing wound healing of critical ischaemic foot after bypass surgery: is the angiosome important in selecting bypass target artery? Eur J Vasc Endovasc Surg 2012;43(3):322–8.

15. Varela C, Acin F, de Haro J, et al. The role of foot collateral vessels on ulcer healing and limb salvage after successful endovascular and surgical distal procedures according to an angiosome model. Vasc Endovascular Surg 2010;44(8):654–60.

16. Rashid H, Slim H, Zayed H, et al. The impact of arterial pedal arch quality and angiosome revascularization on foot tissue loss healing and infrapopliteal bypass outcome. J Vasc Surg 2013;57(5):1219–26.

17. Fernandez N, McEnaney R, Marone LK, et al. Multilevel versus isolated endovascular tibial interventions for critical limb ischemia. J Vasc Surg 2011;54(3):722–9.

18. Castronuovo JJ Jr, Adera HM, Smiell JM, et al. Skin perfusion pressure measurement is valuable in the diagnosis of critical limb ischemia. J Vasc Surg 1997;26(4):629–37.

19. Faris I, Duncan H. Skin perfusion pressure in the prediction of healing in diabetic patients with ulcers or gangrene of the foot. J Vasc Surg 1985;2(4):536–40.

20. Iida O, Nanto S, Uematsu M, et al. Importance of the angiosome concept for endovascular therapy in patients with critical limb ischemia. Catheter Cardiovasc Interv 2010;75(6):830–6.

21. Utsunomiya M, Nakamura M, Nakanishi M, et al. Impact of wound blush as an angiographic end point of endovascular therapy for patients with critical limb ischemia. J Vasc Surg 2012;55(1):113–21.

22. Yamada T, Ohta T, Ishibashi H, et al. Clinical reliability and utility of skin perfusion pressure measurement in ischemic limbs: comparison with other noninvasive diagnostic methods. J Vasc Surg 2008;47(2):318–23.

23. Rother U, Kapust J, Lang W, et al. The angiosome concept evaluated on the basis of microperfusion in critical limb ischemia patients: an Oxygen to See Guided Study. Microcirculation 2015;22(8):737–43.

24. Biancari F, Juvonen T. Angiosome-targeted lower limb revascularization for ischemic foot wounds: systematic review and meta-analysis. Eur J Vasc Endovasc Surg 2014;47(5):517–22.

25. Bosanquet DC, Glasbey JC, Williams IM, et al. Systematic review and meta-analysis of direct versus indirect angiosomal revascularisation of infrapopliteal arteries. Eur J Vasc Endovasc Surg 2014;48(1):88–97.

26. Huang TY, Huang TS, Wang YC, et al. Direct revascularization with the angiosome concept for lower limb ischemia: a systematic review and meta-analysis. Medicine (Baltimore) 2015;94(34):e1427.

27. Sumpio BE, Forsythe RO, Ziegler KR, et al. Clinical implications of the angiosome model in peripheral vascular disease. J Vasc Surg 2013;58(3):814–26.

28. Alexandrescu VA, Hubermont G, Philips Y, et al. Selective primary angioplasty following an angiosome model of reperfusion in the treatment of Wagner 1-4 diabetic foot lesions: practice in a multidisciplinary diabetic limb service. J Endovasc Ther 2008;15(5):580–93.

29. Deguchi J, Kitaoka T, Yamamoto K, et al. Impact of angiosome on treatment of diabetic ischaemic foot with paramalleolar bypass. J Jpn Coll Angiol 2010;50:687–91.

30. Blanes Orti P, Riera Vazquez R, Puigmacia Minguell P, et al. Percutaneous revascularization of specific angiosome in critical limb ischemia. Angiologia 2011;63:11–7.

31. Soderstrom M, Alback A, Biancari F, et al. Angiosome-targeted infrapopliteal endovascular revascularization for treatment of diabetic foot ulcers. J Vasc Surg 2013;57(2):427–35.

32. Kabra A, Suresh KR, Vivekanand V, et al. Outcomes of angiosome and non-angiosome targeted revascularization in critical lower limb ischemia. J Vasc Surg 2013;57(1):44–9.

33. Fossaceca R, Guzzardi G, Cerini P, et al. Endovascular treatment of diabetic foot in a selected population of patients with below-the-knee disease: is the angiosome model effective? Cardiovasc Intervent Radiol 2013;36(3):637–44.

34. Lejay A, Georg Y, Tartaglia E, et al. Long-term outcomes of direct and indirect below-the-knee open revascularization based on the angiosome concept in diabetic patients with critical limb ischemia. Ann Vasc Surg 2014;28(4):983–9.

35. Acin F, Varela C, Lopez de Maturana I, et al. Results of infrapopliteal endovascular procedures performed in diabetic patients with critical limb ischemia and tissue loss from the perspective of an angiosome-oriented revascularization strategy. Int J Vasc Med 2014;2014:270539.

36. Kret MR, Cheng D, Azarbal AF, et al. Utility of direct angiosome revascularization and runoff scores in predicting outcomes in patients undergoing revascularization for critical limb ischemia. J Vasc Surg 2014;59(1):121–8.

37. Spillerova K, Biancari F, Leppaniemi A, et al. Differential impact of bypass surgery and angioplasty on angiosome-targeted infrapopliteal revascularization. Eur J Vasc Endovasc Surg 2015;49(4):412–9.

Emerging and Future Therapeutic Options for Femoropopliteal and Infrapopliteal Endovascular Intervention

Damianos G. Kokkinidis, MD,
Ehrin J. Armstrong, MD, MSc*

KEYWORDS

- Peripheral vascular disease • Drug-eluting stents • Drug-eluting balloons
- Bioresorbable scaffolds • Postangioplasty dissection • Adventitial delivery • Arterial calcification

KEY POINTS

- Emerging endovascular technologies for the treatment of peripheral artery disease promise to improve procedural and patient outcomes.
- New drug-coated balloons, drug-eluting stents, and bioresorbable scaffolds have all shown encouraging initial results for treatment of femoropopliteal disease.
- The Tack-It device, peripheral Lithoplasty, and adventitial delivery of medications are examples of novel technologies that can potentially offer alternative options for the treatment of peripheral artery disease.

INTRODUCTION

Peripheral artery disease (PAD) affects more than 200 million people worldwide.[1,2] Most patients with PAD have lesions that are located in the femoral or popliteal arteries (femoropopliteal [FP] disease), which typically presents as lifestyle-limiting claudication. Infrapopliteal disease (ie, occurring below the knee [BTK]) is particularly common in diabetic patients who have multilevel disease and is associated with critical limb ischemia (CLI).[3,4] The superficial femoral artery (SFA) poses many technical challenges to long-term durability of endovascular interventions: it is one of the longest vessels in the body and actively participates in knee motion, which leads to torsion of the vessel. As a result, many stent-based technologies have historically had limited patency rates for FP disease. BTK lesions also pose several technical challenges. These lesions are usually long, with a smaller vessel diameter and dense calcification, characteristics that complicate their endovascular management. Even if acute success rates are satisfying, restenosis after endovascular procedures is a common limitation encountered with current technologies.[5,6] For both FP and BTK disease, continued innovation has introduced new devices, techniques, and treatment combinations (Table 1). This article summarizes the emerging and future endovascular technologies for the treatment of FP and BTK arteries.

Disclosures: D.G. Kokkinidis reports no conflicts of interest. E.J. Armstrong is a consultant/advisory board member for Abbott Vascular, Boston Scientific, Cardiovascular Systems, Medtronic, and Spectranetics.
Section of Cardiology, Denver VA Medical Center, University of Colorado School of Medicine, 1055 Clermont Street, Denver, CO 80220, USA
* Corresponding author.
E-mail address: Ehrin.armstrong@gmail.com

Table 1
Summary of novel technologies for the treatment of peripheral artery disease

Study	Novel Technology or Approach	Study Design Study Location	PAD Location Enrollment (n) Comparison	Primary End Points	Announced or Published Results	Other Studies on the Same Technology
REALITY (NCT02850107)	HawkOne or TurboHawk and the IN.PACT Admiral DCB	Multicenter, prospective, single-arm study USA	FP 250 (–)	• Freedom from 12-m PP and CD-TLR • Freedom from 30-d MAE	(–)	DEFINITE AR
ILLUMENATE Global registry (NCT01927068)	Stellarex DCB	Multicenter, prospective, single-arm study Europe, Australia, New Zealand	FP 501 (–)	• Freedom from 30-d device and procedure-related mortality • Freedom from 12-m TLMA and CD-TLR • 12-m PP	1-y PP: 84.7% Freedom from 12-m CD-TLR: 91%	ILLUMENATE studies: pivotal, FIH, PK, and European randomized trial
RANGER-SFA (NCT02013193)	Ranger DCB	Multicenter, prospective, randomized study Europe	FP 105 Uncoated BA	6-m LLL (in-segment)	6-m TLR: 5.6% (Ranger) vs 12% (BA)	Ranger DCB studies: all-comers registry, Ranger BTK, COMPARE I pilot treatment study (Ranger vs IN.PACT DCB, n = 150)
EffPac (NCT02540018)	Luminor 35 DCB	Multicenter, prospective, randomized controlled study Germany	SFA 172 Uncoated BA	6-m and 12-m LLL	(–)	(–)
MAJESTIC (NCT02013193)	ELUVIA nitinol self-expanding PES	Multicenter, prospective, single-arm study Europe, Australia, New Zealand	FP 57 (–)	9-m PP	Technical success: 97% Freedom from 12-m TLR: 96.5%	IMPERIAL Study (Eluvia vs Zilver PES Stent, n>450)
ESPIRIT I (NCT01468974)	ESPIRIT BVS	Multicenter, prospective, single-arm, FIH trial Europe	SFA/iliac 35 (–)	• Device success • Technical success • Clinical success [a]No primary end point	Procedural success: 100% 1-y, 2-y, and 3-y TLR: 8.8%, 11.8%, and 11.8%	(–)

Study	Intervention	Study Design	Vessel / N / Comparator	Endpoints	Results	Comments
SPRINT (NCT02097082)	480 Biomedical Stanza drug-eluting BVS	Multicenter, prospective, single-arm study Europe and New Zealand	SFA; NA; (—)	• 6-m DUS patency (defined as ≤50% restenosis) • 30-d MAE	(—)	(—)	STANCE trial
DESappear Study (NCT02869087)	Akesys Prava BVS	Multicenter, prospective, single-arm study Europe and New Zealand	SFA; 60; (—)	• Freedom from the composite end point of 30-d POD and 6-m MALE • 6-m PP	(—)	(—)
Varcoe et al,[52,98] 2015 and 2016 (Absorb BVS for BTK)	Absorb BVS	Safety and feasibility single-center study Australia	BTK; 14; (—)	• CV and all-cause mortality • 30-d LLL, TLBPS, and TLR • Technical success	Freedom from CD-TLR at 12 and 24 m: 96% 12 and 24-m KM (Kaplan-Meier) curves estimate for PP 96% and 84.6%	The ABSORB Bioresorbable Scaffold BTK Study (n = 60)
DANCE (NCT01983449)	Bullfrog Micro-Infusion Device for adventitial dexamethasone delivery	Multicenter, prospective, single-arm study United States	FP; 281 (157 and 124); (—)	• 6-m and 12-m binary restenosis (DUS) • 30-d MALE+POD	395-d PP and freedom from TLR: 76.6% and 89%	(—)
LIMBO (NCT02479555 and NCT02479620)	Bullfrog Micro-Infusion device for adventitial dexamethasone delivery	Multicenter, prospective, randomized pilot studies Europe and USA	BTK; 120 each; angioplasty without dexamethasone delivery	• 6-m freedom from MALE, CD-TLR • 6-m TVAL% change • Composite of freedom from 30-d death and 6-m MALE, amputations or CD-TLR	(—)	(—)
TANGO (NCT02908035)	Adventitial delivery of temsirolimus (Torisel)	Multicenter, prospective, randomized study United States	BTK (CLI); 60; Saline delivery	• 30-d freedom from MALE-POD • 6-m TVAL%	(—)	(—)

(continued on next page)

Study	Novel Technology or Approach	Study Design Study Location	PAD Location Enrollment (n) Comparison	Primary End Points	Announced or Published Results	Other Studies on the Same Technology
Pilot study of PRT-201 following BA in patients with PAD	Adventitial delivery of PRT-201 (vonapanitase)	Phase I study United States	FP 14 (−)	12-m clinical safety	(−)	(−)
TOBA (NCT01663818)	Tack Endovascular System	Multicenter, prospective, single-arm, post-CE mark study Europe	FP 130 (−)	30-d Composite of all new-onset device-related MAE	Technical success: 98.5% 12-m patency: 76.4% 12-m freedom from TLR: 89.5%	TOBA II, TOBA III, TOBA-BTK
DISRPUT PAD (NCT02071108, NCT01577888)	Shockwave Lithoplasty	Multicenter, prospective, single-arm study Europe and New Zealand	FP 95 (−)	• 30-d MAE freedom • Procedural success	Procedural success[b]: 89.5% 6-m patency: 77% 6-m TLR: 3.2%	Disrupt PAD III (Lithoplasty with DCB vs DCB alone, n = 300) safety and feasibility of Lithoplasty BTK

Abbreviations: ATK, above the knee; BA, Balloon angioplasty; BTK, below the knee; BVS, bioresorbable vascular scaffolds; CD-TLR, clinical driven–target lesion revascularization; CE, Conformité Européene; CLI, critical limb ischemia; CV, cardiovascular; DCB, drug-coated balloons; DUS, duplex ultrasonography; FIH, first in human; FP, femoropopliteal; LLL, late lumen loss; MAE, major adverse events; MALE-POD, major adverse limb events–perioperative death; PES, paclitaxel-eluting stent; PK, pharmacokinetics; PP, primary patency; SFA, superficial femoral artery; TLBPS, target lesion bypass surgery; TLMA, target limb major amputation; TVAL%, transverse-view vessel area loss percentage.

[a] For more detailed definitions of the end points, visit individual study protocols at clinicaltrials.gov.

[b] Defined as residual stenosis less than 30%.

NOVEL DRUG-COATED BALLOONS

Drug-coated balloons (DCB) and drug-eluting stents (DESs) inhibit the proliferation of smooth muscle cells that contribute to neointimal hyperplasia and restenosis. Current DCB are coated with paclitaxel at a concentration between 2 and 3.5 $\mu g/mm^2$. Paclitaxel has lipophilic properties that enable its absorption into the arterial wall, thereby leading to retention of drug in the vessel wall.[7] More than 10 DCB are Conformité Européene (CE) marked and available in Europe but only 2 are currently US Food and Drug Administration (FDA) approved for use in the United States. DCB systems differ in the details of the coated technology used and in their excipients: iopromide (Paccocath), citric acid ester (Ranger), dextran,[8] urea (IN.PACT), shellac (Freeway), butyryl trihexyl citrate (BIO-LUX), polysorbate/sorbitol (Lutonix), polyethylene glycol (Stellarex), resveratrol (Sequent Please OTW), or none. The excipient and proprietary coating technology used in a given DCB likely influences paclitaxel delivery and clinical outcomes among these devices.

Drug-coated Balloons for Femoropopliteal Disease

DCB are superior to conventional balloon angioplasty (BA) for treatment of FP lesions of moderate length, with excellent primary patency rates.[9-11] In a recent prospective registry that included longer (>150 mm) SFA lesions and real-world patients, the 12-month primary patency rate was 83% with a clinically driven (CD) target lesion revascularization (TLR) rate of 4%.[12] There are some published data supporting that DCB, when used in SFA, result in similar, if not superior, patency rates compared with stenting. However, published comparisons have not yet shown a clear superiority of DCB compared with DES.[13-15]

Drug-coated Balloons for Infrapopliteal Disease

Although DCB are highly effective for the treatment of FP lesions, trials to date have not shown a benefit of DCB for treatment of infrapopliteal PAD.[16-19] The few trials that have indicated superiority for infrapopliteal DCB were single center,[17-19] whereas multicenter trials failed to confirm these results.[16,20] A single-center retrospective study that used the Lutonix DCB reported a TLR rate of 15.9% and a major amputation rate of 4.1% over a median follow-up of 9 months.[21] Recently, the Biotronik Passeo-18 LUX DCB was compared with the uncoated Passeo-18 percutaneous transluminal angioplasty (PTA) balloon in patients requiring revascularization of infrapopliteal arteries (BIOLUX P-II trial).[20] This first-in-human (FIH) study showed that this DCB is safe and effective for treatment of infrapopliteal lesions compared with PTA (the primary safety end point was 0% in the DCB group vs 8.3% in the PTA group; $P = .239$). A study in Sweden is currently enrolling patients to compare DCB with PTA for crural arteries in 70 patients, testing the primary patency 12 months after the procedure (NCT02750605).

Novel Drug-coated Balloon Technologies and Approaches

The aim of new DCB technologies is to reduce drug loss during balloon inflation and to increase the deliverability and absorption of drug from the arterial walls. Apart from emerging devices, newer studies are also investigating the possible benefit of combining plaque modification with DCB angioplasty. The combination of atherectomy and DCB compared with DCB alone for long BTK lesions is being studied in a single-center, prospective, randomized study in Germany that will enroll 80 patients (NCT01763476). The primary end point is the in-segment binary restenosis at 3-month postprocedural angiographic follow-up. Similarly, the DEFINITIVE AR study is a multicenter, prospective, randomized study that compared the potential benefit of directional atherectomy (DA) use before the Cotavance DCB. Results showed that atherectomy and DCB group 12-month primary patency rates for severely calcified lesions treated were 70.4% versus 62.5% for patients treated with DCB alone (Zeller T. Vascular InterVentional Advances 2014, Las Vegas, NV). Another ongoing study is the multicenter, prospective, single-arm REALITY Study (directional atherectomy and DCB to treat long, calcified FP artery stenosis), where in which Medtronic's DA systems (Medtronic HawkOne or Medtronic TurboHawk) and the IN.PACT Admiral DCB will be studied in 250 patients. Twelve-month and 24-month follow-up will assess primary patency and CD-TLR respectively (NCT02850107).

Stellarex drug-coated balloon

The Stellarex DCB (Spectranetics Corporation) uses a proprietary EnduraCoat coating technology. The paclitaxel concentration of the balloon surface is 2 $\mu g/mm^2$, and the excipient used is polyethylene glycol. Stellarex received the CE mark in December 2014. Five different studies are designed to assess the Stellarex DCB: ILLUMENATE Pivotal (NCT01858428), ILLUMENATE FIH,[22] ILLUMENATE pharmacokinetic

(NCT01912937), ILLUMENATE European Randomized Trial (NCT01858363), and ILLUMENATE Global registry (NCT01927068). The ILLUMENATE Global registry, a multicenter, prospective single-arm study for treatment of FP lesions, recently reported 12-month follow-up data (Zeller T. Charing Cross Symposium 2016, London, United Kingdom). The mean lesion length in this study was 7.3 cm, with 42.4% calcified vessels and 25.6% chronic total occlusions. The 1-year primary patency was 84.7% (89.5% and 80.3% for 12-month and 24-month follow-up respectively in the ILLUMENATE FIH) and the freedom from CD-TLR was 91% (90% and 85.8% for 12-month and 24-month follow-up respectively in the ILLUMENATE pharmacokinetic study). The ILLUMENATE European RCT enrolled 328 patients and randomized 295 subjects to Stellarex DCB or conventional BA. Kaplan-Meier estimates for primary patency were 89% for the DCB group versus 65% for BA, and Kaplan-Meier estimates for freedom from CD-TLR were 94.8% for the DCB group and 85.3% for the PTA group (Brodmann M, Amputation Prevention Symposium 2016, Chicago, IL). The ILLUMENATE Pivotal study 1-year results were also recently reported. For the primary safety end point (composite of 30-day freedom from device-related and procedure-related death, and the 12-month freedom from target limb major amputation and CD-TLR) Stellarex was superior to BA (92.1% vs 83.2%; $P = .001$). The primary effectiveness end point was defined as a composite of absence of restenosis (identified with DUS) and freedom from CD-TLR at 12-month follow-up. Stellarex was superior to BA (76.3% vs 57.6%; $P = .003$). The 365-day primary patency rate was 82.3% for DCB versus 70.9% for BA (Lyden S, Transcatheter Cardiovascular Therapeutics 2016, Washington DC).

Ranger drug-coated balloon
The Ranger DCB (Boston Scientific Corporation) uses a proprietary TransPax coating system. A citrate ester excipient leads to a novel hydrophobic form of paclitaxel and enables an improved deliverability, stability (potentially decreasing embolization risk), and efficacy, and a sustained release of paclitaxel. The comparison between the Ranger DCB and conventional BA for FP lesions from a multicenter RCT with 105 patients (Ranger-SFA) showed that the Ranger was superior in 6-month TLR: 5.6% versus 12% for BA (Scheinert D, Cardiovascular and Interventional Radiology Society of Europe 2016, Barcelona). Follow-up will continue up to 3 years (NCT02013193). An additional study on

the Ranger DCB for FP lesion is an all-comer registry with 180 patients (NCT02462005). The primary safety end point is defined as major adverse events (MAE), a composite of device-related and procedure-related mortality and major limb amputation after 6 months, and the primary efficacy end point as 12-month and 24-month primary patency. The 6-month results showed a Kaplan-Meier estimate for primary patency of 91.1%, whereas the freedom from TLR was 91.9% (Von Bilderling, Cardiovascular and Interventional Radiology Society of Europe 2016, Barcelona). Ranger DCB will be also evaluated by (1) RANGER BTK in France, with 30 patients with BTK lesions (NCT02856230); (2) COMPARE I pilot treatment study, which will compare the Ranger DCB versus the IN.PACT DCB in 150 patients (NCT02701543).

Luminor drug-coated balloon
The paclitaxel-coated balloon Luminor 35 (iVascular, SLU, Barcelona, Spain) uses the coating technology Transfertech with a paclitaxel dose of 3 μg/mm^2 and can be used for both FP and BTK disease. The balloon is coated with paclitaxel and a physiologically innocuous matrix. In a preclinical swine model, this DCB reduced in-stent restenosis (ISR) compared with BA.[23] A phase-III multicenter RCT is being conducted in Germany (172 patients) to assess the effectiveness of the Luminor balloon in the SFA compared with BA (NCT02540018). The primary end point is 6-month and 12-month late lumen loss.

NOVEL DRUG-ELUTING STENTS
Drug-eluting Stents for Femoropopliteal Disease
Although published trials have shown that the use of a nitinol self-expanding stent instead of conventional BA was associated with improved outcomes,[24] and despite recent advancements in stent technology, the increasing pressure to the FP axis caused by walking and sitting leads to a higher risk of stent fracture and subsequent ISR.[25–28] At the same time, drug-eluting nitinol stents have been proved superior to primary nitinol stenting and BA for SFA treatment, albeit with older-generation nitinol stents. The Zilver paclitaxel-eluting stent (Zilver PTX) is a self-expanding nitinol DES with a polymer-free paclitaxel coating. Many trials and real-world studies have investigated Zilver PTX and proved it to be superior to BA with provisional Bare-metal stent (BMS) for patients with FP disease. Two-year results showed an improved survival and primary patency for the Zilver PTX group compared with BA with provisional stenting.[29] Five-year results

confirmed the effectiveness and safety of the Zilver in terms of freedom from TLR and patency.[30] With respect to provisional stenting, DES was superior to BMS. Recent studies have expanded those results in real-world populations.[31]

Drug-eluting Stents for Infrapopliteal Disease

Considering that BTK disease is often associated with CLI, the primary goal of revascularization for BTK intervention is to prolong amputation-free survival.[32] BTK vessels tend to have a smaller diameter and a poorer run-off. These characteristics, combined with a lack of specialized endovascular technology, have been associated with lower rates of patency compared with FP disease.[33] At present, the short-term results for BTK angioplasty are encouraging but long-term patency and clinical improvement remain unsolved problems.[34,35] Published trials, with the exception of the PADI (Percutaneous Transluminal Angioplasty and Drug-Eluting Stents for Infrapopliteal Lesions in Critical Limb Ischemia) study,[36] did not result in a significant clinical improvement or an increase in the amputation-free survival, but DES were still superior to BA and BMS from an angiographic standpoint.[37–39] Although the IDEAS (Infrapopliteal Drug-Eluting Angioplasty Versus Stenting) study showed that DES can be also used for longer lesions and resulted in lower 6-month restenosis rates compared with DCB,[40] current recommendations support DES use only for focal and proximal lesions of the tibial artery as a bailout strategy.

Novel Drug-eluting Stents

Eluvia drug-eluting stent

The Eluvia stent uses the Innova self-expanding nitinol stent system platform. It has a sustained drug release with more than 90% being released over 1 year. The stent coating system consists of a primer layer of poly n-butyl methacrylate (PBMA), whereas the active layer is composed of the fluoropolymer poly(vinylidene fluoride-co-hexafluoropropylene) and paclitaxel.[41] Contrary to what occurs in the coronary arteries, paclitaxel may be more effective than –limus drugs for treatment of SFA atherosclerotic disease. MAJESTIC, a prospective, single-arm study, enrolled 57 patients with SFA or proximal popliteal lesions less than 110 mm treated with Eluvia and reported that only 2 patients underwent TLR at 1-year follow-up.[42]

Results from preclinical and clinical trials showed that the combination of the Eluvia polymer with paclitaxel can result in a clinically meaningful antirestenotic effect and a lower rate of neointimal proliferation after 90 days compared with BMS.

The IMPERIAL Study is a randomized single-blind study that will enroll more than 450 patients. This study will compare Eluvia with the Zilver PTX stent (NCT02574481), resulting in the first head-to-head comparison of DES for treatment FP disease.

BIORESORBABLE SCAFFOLDS

Balloon-expandable DES and thin-strut nitinol stents used for treatment of PAD have reduced rates of ISR, but placement of a permanent scaffold has inherent limitations, including the long-term risk of restenosis. The introduction of bioresorbable vascular scaffolds (BVS) has the potential to revolutionize interventional cardiology. BVS provide initial structural support for the arterial wall but are then absorbed over the course of 2 to 3 years, thereby minimizing inflammatory or allergic reactions and the risk of stent fracture.[43–45] Scaffold absorption also enables the future use of imaging techniques such as magnetic resonance angiography and increases convenience regarding the possible need of future endovascular procedures or surgeries. However, BVS degradation time with available technologies has not yet been optimized to balance scaffold support with minimization of inflammatory risk.[46] Diabetics and elderly patients represent the most common population with PAD and have higher rates of vascular calcification and long BTK lesions. Lesions such as these are not ideal candidates for BVS with currently available technology. Moreover, the next generation of nitinol stents for FP lesions and balloon-expandable metallic stents for BTK lesions offer excellent alternative options that might be superior to BVS. Future expectations from BVS include newer mechanical properties resembling expandable stents and smaller size of scaffolds.

The balloon-expandable bare (ie, non–drug-eluting) Igaki-Tamai stent (Remedy, Kyoto Medical Planning, Kyoto, Japan) is the first BVS that was used for the SFA. It was tested in the PERSEUS (Prospective Evaluation in a Randomized Trial of the Safety and Efficacy of the Use of the TAXUS Element Paclitaxel-Eluting Coronary Stent System) trial, achieving 100% technical success but the 12-month patency rates were only 50%.[47] Recently, results from a real-world registry with short FP lesions, which tested the REMEDY BVS, were announced. Twelve-month primary patency rates were 58%, again less than the rates that can be achieved with the use of modern nitinol stents.[48] A future trial is planned to investigate the drug-coated REMEDY stent (Kyoto Medical Planning Co.), an improved version of the Igaki-Tamai scaffold, with increased stent strength and an antiproliferative coating. The use of DCB before Igaki-Tamai scaffold was evaluated in 20 patients in the GAIA-DEB study, decreasing the average percentage of diameter stenosis.[49]

BVS have been tested in the past for infrapopliteal lesions. The Biotronik bioabsorbable magnesium-alloy stent was the first BVS that was safely implanted in BTK arteries.[47,50,51] The absorbable metal stent (AMS) balloon-expandable stent (Biotronik, Berlin, Germany), which is made of magnesium, zirconium, yttrium, and other elements, was tested in 117 patients with CLI in the AMS INSIGHT (Bioabsorbable Metal Stent Investigation in Chronic Limb Ischemia Treatment) trial. Patients were treated with either AMS stenting or BA for focal infrapopliteal lesions less than 15 mm.[46] The results were not satisfying, with clearly worse 6-month primary patency rates (32% vs 58%; $P = .013$) for the AMS group, probably caused by its fast absorption (almost 4 months) and imperfect mechanical properties.

Drug-Eluting Bioresorbable Vascular Scaffold for Femoropopliteal Disease
ESPRIT bioresorbable vascular scaffold
The ESPRIT I is a multicenter, prospective, single-arm, FIH trial that evaluated the Esprit BVS in 35 symptomatic SFA or iliac atherosclerotic lesions (NCT01468974). The Esprit BVS consists of an everolimus-eluting PLLA (poly-Llactide) scaffold. The procedural success rate was 100% and no scaffold recoils or binary restenosis were reported acutely or in 30-day duplex follow-up respectively. After 2 years, there was 1 death (unrelated) but no amputations. The TLR rate was 8.8% after 1 year and 11.8% after 2 years. Recently, the ESPIRIT I Trial's 3-year results were announced, confirming and expanding to 3 years the safety and feasibility of Esprit BVS for SFA and iliac lesions (Jaff M, Vascular Interventional Advances 2016, Las Vegas, NV). No new events occurred between 2 and 3 years.

480 Biomedical stanza drug-eluting bioresorbable vascular scaffold
The SPRINT trial is an ongoing study evaluating the 480 Biomedical Stanza BVS in patients with SFA disease. The primary outcomes are (1) 6-month patency and (2) MAE after 30 days (Holden A, Charing Cross International Symposium 2014, London). The estimated enrollment is 70 patients (NCT02097082). Before the SPRINT trial, the STANCE (An Evaluation of the 480 Biomedical STANZA Drug-Eluting Resorbable Scaffold [DRS] System in the Treatment of de novo SFA Lesions) trial, a multicenter,

prospective, single-arm, FIH study, tested the 480 Biomedical Stanza BVS for SFA lesions less than 100 mm in 46 patients (NCT01403077). This technology was similar to the one that will be tested in the SPRINT trial, but without drug-eluting properties. Stanza is a self-expanding stent with a polylactic-co-glycolic acid and bioresorbable elastomer composite. When tested in animals, a biocompatible resorption of the scaffold over 6 to 12 months was shown.

Akesys Prava sirolimus-eluting bioresorbable vascular scaffold
The DESappear study (Drug-Eluting Scaffold with an Absorbable Platform for Primary Lower Extremity Arterial Revascularization) is a multicenter prospective single-arm study that will test the safety and effectiveness of the Prava sirolimus-eluting bioresorbable scaffold system for the treatment of 60 patients with SFA disease. The first BVS was recently successfully implanted. Patients will have a clinical follow-up at 1, 6, 12, 24, and 36 months after the implantation of the Prava BVS, and primary patency (primary effectiveness outcome) is defined as 6-month freedom from CD-TLR or greater than 50% lesion diameter reduction (NCT02869087).

Drug-Eluting Bioresorbable Vascular Scaffold for Infrapopliteal Disease
Everolimus-eluting BVS for infrapopliteal arteries had been tested in the past in the ABSORB BTK multicenter, single-arm trial (NCT01341340), but the study was terminated because of poor enrollment. The Absorb BVS has similar mechanical and antiproliferative properties to the newer-generation DES and is hydrolyzed and absorbed over the course of 3 years.[52] Varcoe and colleagues[52] implanted 22 Absorb BVS in 18 lesions, with an initial technical success rate of 100%. No binary restenosis, amputation, or bypass surgery patient deaths were reported in the follow-up (6.1 ± 3.9 months), whereas clinical improvement was seen in 12 patients (including 4 with CLI). During 12-month follow-up, freedom from CD-TLR was 96%, whereas the Kaplan-Meier estimate for primary patency was 96%, 96%, and 84.6% after 6, 12, and 24 months. These initial promising results have led to discussion of a possible randomized study to investigate the efficacy of the Absorb BVS for treatment of infrapopliteal lesions. Fig. 1 shows a patient with CLI and infrapopliteal disease who was treated with bioresorbable scaffold implantation.

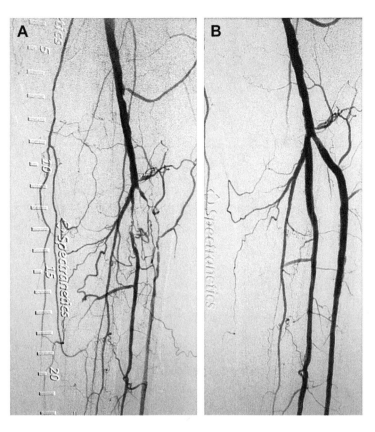

Fig. 1. Bioresorbable scaffold implantation for infrapopliteal peripheral artery disease. A 69-year-old man presented with a nonhealing wound of his left great toe. (A) Lower extremity angiography revealed subtotal occlusion of the proximal anterior tibial artery and severe stenosis at the origin of the peroneal artery. (B) Angiographic result after implantation of two 3.5 × 28 mm everolimus-eluting bioresorbable scaffolds in the anterior tibial artery, and one 3.0 × 28 mm bioresorbable scaffold in the peroneal artery.

PERIVASCULAR OR ADVENTITIAL DELIVERY OF DRUGS TO LIMIT RESTENOSIS

The adventitia, the outer layer of an arterial vessel, offers a unique environment to achieve maximum drug concentration,[53] and has been shown to contribute to inflammatory reactions after angioplasty. Most of the fibroblasts that lead to restenosis originate from the adventitia and migrate toward the intima after the balloon injury.[54–59] Thus, perivascular or adventitial drug delivery represents a novel potential mechanism to improve outcomes after endovascular intervention.

Dexamethasone, a broad-spectrum antiinflammatory agent, can effectively block this cascade. Owens and colleagues,[60] in a single-center, prospective, investigator-initiated study, used the Bullfrog Micro-Infusion Catheter (Mercator MedSystems, San Leandro, CA) to inject dexamethasone directly to the adventitia of the SFA. The Bullfrog catheter is FDA 510(k)–cleared for use in coronary and peripheral arteries. When the balloon is inflated, a needle directed toward the vessel wall penetrates the vessel wall and delivers infusate and contrast (4:1) into the adventitia. Mixing of contrast with the infusate ensures that the infusate is retained in the vessel wall, rather than the bloodstream. In an FIH study, 3.0 ± 1.3 injections were required per centimeter, whereas the mean volume injected was 3.8 ± 1.9 mL; no amputations, death, device-related adverse events, or binary restenosis occurred during 6-month follow-up. After this preliminary FIH trial, the DANCE (The Delivery of Dexamethasone to the Adventitia to eNhance Clinical Efficacy after Femoropopliteal Revascularization) trial was the next to investigate the Bullfrog device. DANCE is a multicenter, single-arm trial that enrolled 281 patients (NCT01983449). Patients were treated with either atherectomy (157 patients) or PTA (124 patients) and with dexamethasone adventitial infusion, at a dose of 1.6 mg/cm. The primary efficacy end point for this study was the 12-month primary patency (79.5% according to Kaplan-Meier), defined as lack of TLR and duplex ultrasonography peak systolic velocity ratio less than or equal to 2.4. At 12-month follow-up the rates for TLR, SAE (device and drug related), amputations, and death were 89.7%, 0%, 0.6%, and 5.1%

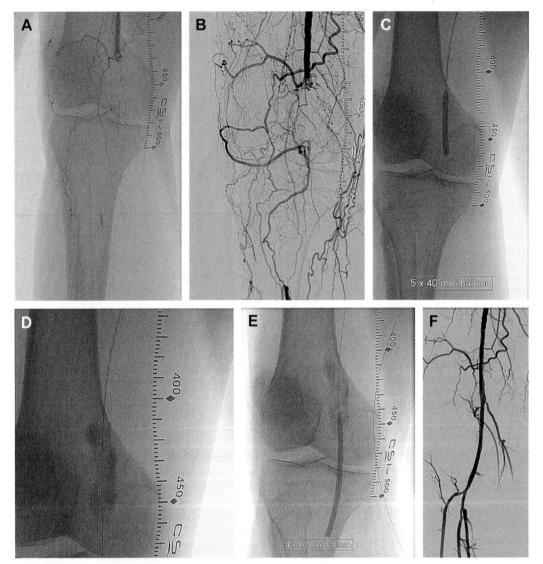

Fig. 2. Adventitial delivery of dexamethasone to treat peripheral artery disease. A 72-year-old man presented with severe lifestyle-limiting claudication despite maximal medical therapy and a walking program. (A) Lower extremity angiography revealed an occluded popliteal artery. (B) Subtracted image shows reconstitution in the distal popliteal artery segment. (C) The lesion was crossed and initial angioplasty performed. (D) A Bullfrog device was used to infuse dexamethasone into the adventitial space. Mixing of the drug with dilute contrast confirms adventitial delivery. (E) Further balloon angioplasty was performed. (F) Final angiographic result.

respectively. Combined results for the atherectomy and PTA groups after a follow-up period of 395 days showed primary patency and freedom from TLR rates of 76.6% and 89% respectively (Owens C, Vascular InterVentional Advances 2016, Las Vegas, NV). Fig. 2 shows a patient with severe claudication and a popliteal artery occlusion who was treated with BA followed by adventitial infusion of dexamethasone.

Two more trials are currently investigating the feasibility and effectiveness of the Bullfrog device for the treatment of patients with CLI caused by BTK disease. The LIMBO (Lower-Limb Adventitial Infusion of DexaMet hasone Via Bullfrog to Reduce Occurrence of Restenosis) trials are 2 multicenter, prospective, randomized, pilot studies that are enrolling patients in Europe (NCT02479555) and the United States (NCT02479620) to test dexamethasone administration (4 mg/mL) with PTA and atherectomy respectively. Each trial will include up to 120 patients (60 treated with dexamethasone and 60 controls). Adventitial delivery will also be tested for additional restenotic agents. The TANGO (Temsirolimus Adventitial Delivery to Improve Angiographic Outcomes Below the Knee) trial is a multicenter, prospective, randomized, dose-escalation study that will start in 2017 and will document the effects of adventitial delivery of temsirolimus for patients with CLI caused by BTK lesions (NCT02908035). The study will be conducted in 15 centers in the United States and will enroll 60 patients (20 low dose, 20 high dose, and 20 controls). Of note, Nab-rapamycin and paclitaxel adventitial delivery have also already been tested in animal models.[61]

After tibial artery BA, elastic recoil can lead to a loss of 30% of the lumen diameter.[62,63] Under normal circumstances, elastin, a hydrophobic protein that is a fiber and a component of the extracellular matrix, constrains the arterial diameter.[64] Elastase can fragment and remove elastin from selected segments of arteries, resulting in local and permanent dilatation of the treated segment. PRT-201 (Vonapanitase), a recombinant human type1 pancreatic elastase (alternative name: chymotrypsinlike elastase family member 1), is a novel drug candidate for PAD that acts as a vasodilator and can improve blood flow. In blood, alpha1-antitrypsin and alpha2-macroglobulin inactivate elastase,[65] so PRT-201 has to be delivered into the external surface or vessel wall of the blood vessels. Proteon Therapeutics has evaluated adventitial delivery of PRT-201 with a Bullfrog device after BA for FP arteries in a phase-I clinical trial (NCT01616290). Considering the reduction in elastin concentration, aneurysms are an anticipated potential adverse effect and have been reported in porcine arteries models, but without confirmation from clinical studies.[66–68] When used in clinical trials for hemodialysis patients with arteriovenous fistulas and grafts, vonapanitase was proved safe in humans also.[66–68]

MECHANISMS TO LIMIT POSTANGIOPLASTY DISSECTION

Post-PTA dissections present as longitudinal tears and/or flow disturbance in the vessel wall that are visible on angiography. Acute dissection rates after PTA for PAD occur from 47% to 88% of the time.[69,70] Lesions with dissections have a TLR rate 3.5-fold higher compared with lesions without.[69,71] Tepe and colleagues[69] showed that grade C to E dissections had a TLR rate of 44% compared with 33% and 10% for patients with A to B dissections and without dissections, respectively. The dissection flap can be protected with the placement of a stent, and represents one of the main reasons for postangioplasty stent

implantation. In the DCB era, dissections seem to have more favorable outcomes compared with conventional BA, and stent placement is not always necessary,[69] considering that stents can lead to inflammatory reactions, intima hyperplasia, and increased amount of scaffolding in the FP axis, leading eventually to an increased risk of ISR, stent fracture, or even occlusion of the artery.[72,73]

These limitations of stents have led to a demand for more suitable devices for treatment of post-PTA dissections that can fix the dissection and assist in apposition of the tissue, without excessive neointimal hyperplasia and inflammatory reactions. The Tack-It device (Intact Vascular, Inc., Wayne, PA), with a length less than 6 mm and an open lattice design, has 81% less total metal surface and avoids some classic disadvantages of stents but can still be implanted, maintain scaffolding, and potentiate the opposition of the dissection flaps. These characteristics make the Tack-It suitable for different diameters and vessels.

Schneider and colleagues[74] first evaluated the Tack-It device in 25 lesions (6 occlusions) in SFA and popliteal and tibial arteries (average lesion length of 5.6 ± 4.2 cm), with 100% technical success and treatment of all the dissection flaps. At 1-year follow-up, the angiographic patency was 83.3% and restenosis occurred in 16.7% of the lesions. In conjunction with the FIH study, an experimental evaluation was conducted, showing that, at 28-day follow-up, the Tack-It device led to a reduced neointimal proliferation, inflammation, and stenosis rate compared with a self-expanding nitinol stent. After this FIH study, Bosiers and colleagues[75] published results on the Tack Endovascular System (Intact Vascular, Wayne, PA). An average of 3.7 ± 2.1 tacks were used per patient and technical success was achieved in 128 out of 130 patients, with only 2 patients receiving bailout stenting. At 12-month follow-up, the freedom from MAE and TLR was 88% and 89.5% respectively and the primary patency rate was 76.4%. Although lesions longer than 10 cm were not included, Tack-It has the potential to treat multiple dissections with a single device. More TOBA (Tack Optimized Balloon Angioplasty) studies are ongoing. The TOBA II study is investigating the Tack-It in FP disease (NCT02522884). The TOBA III study will include lesions between 20 and 150 mm but also has a subgroup with lesions between 150 and 250 mm (NCT02802306). TOBA-BTK will enroll patients with infrapopliteal lesions and will provide additional clinical data on the outcomes with this device (NCT02235675).

TREATMENT OF PERIPHERAL ARTERY CALCIFICATION

PAD is associated with medial calcification, which is known to increase in more distal parts of the limb.[76,77] Age and cardiovascular risk factors accelerate the progression of calcification.[78] Calcified vessels are associated with higher amputation rates and mortality risk[79,80] and are an obstacle for medication absorption, balloon dilation, and wire crossing.[81] Vessel calcification is also associated with higher risk of recoil after BA, stent fracture, chronic total occlusion, dissection, and embolization.[82–84] For these reasons, RCTs of novel endovascular devices usually exclude calcified lesions.

Atherectomy devices can be combined with BA or stenting and have been shown to be effective for the management of calcified vessels. The idea behind these devices is based on the potential to reduce calcification and improve lesion compliance, enabling interventionalists to place balloons and stents with greater convenience.[85] There are 4 different methods available: orbital atherectomy, DA, rotational atherectomy (RA), and laser atherectomy.

Orbital atherectomy includes the CSI Diamondback Orbital atherectomy system (Cardiovascular Systems, Inc.). This device has a diamond-coated abrasive crown (Diamondback) that rotates at high speed and can be used for calcified and fibrotic plaques, and has the ability to selectively remove calcium,[86] improving BA procedural success and minimizing the need for bailout stenting,[87] thus leading to lower TLR rates.[88] DA includes the SilverHawk, TurboHawk, and HawkOne devices and can be combined with distal embolic protection devices such as the SpiderFX embolic protection filter (Covidien) as in the DEFINITE CA (Directional AthErectomy Followed by a PaclItaxel-Coated BallooN to InhibiT RestenosIs and Maintain Vessel PatEncy: A Pilot Study of Anti-Restenosis Treatment) registry (NCT01366482). In the TALON (Treating Peripherals With SilverHawk: Outcomes Collection) registry, the SilverHawk device was used in addition to provisional PTA or stenting. Minko and colleagues[89] reported a primary patency rate of 69% in 1-year follow-up after the use of the SilverHawk device for FP lesions. RA includes the Jetstream (Boston Scientific), the Rotoblator (Boston Scientific), and the Phoenix atherectomy (AtheroMed) devices. RA devices act by removing superficial calcium from FP lesions, enabling the proper expansion of the adjunctive balloon and stent. RA was tested in 172 patients, with half of them having moderate to high levels of calcification, and led to a TLR rate of 26%.[90] The Jetstream G3 calcium device is currently being tested and has been proved to adequately detect and remove calcium with low TLR rates.[91] Moreover, the concomitant use of a distal filter device can reduce embolization rates.[92] The CliRpath Excimer Laser System to Enlarge Lumen Openings single-arm study evaluated the use of laser atherectomy and found that the freedom of TLR was 76.9% at 12-month follow-up.[93] Atherectomy can also be combined with DCB (IN.PACT Admiral). In a small study by Cioppa and colleagues,[94] it was shown that the combination of the TurboHawk and DCB with a distal protection device (SpiderFX) can lower the bailout stenting rates and the 12-month primary patency. The freedom from TLR after 1 year was 90%.

Novel Treatments for Peripheral Calcification

Many attempts to improve the available technology for peripheral calcification have been conducted. Khalid and colleagues[95] used a high-frequency vibration energy catheter (CROSSER, Bard Peripheral Vascular Inc., Tempe, AZ), whereas Spaargaren and colleagues[81] reported a high success rate using a balloon catheter that has enhanced ability to be pushed. According to the PIERCE (percutaneous direct needle puncture of calcified plaque) technique, a needle crack to the calcified wall can help the catheter tip to be unlocked and advanced through the vessel, while permitting balloon passage and dilation.[96]

Lithoplasty for Treatment of Calcified Lesions

Recently the 6-month results of the DISRPUT PAD study (NCT02071108 and NCT02369848) were announced (Zeller T, Vascular InterVentional Advances 2016, Las Vegas, NV). The DISRUPT PAD (Safety and Performance Study of the Shockwave Lithoplasty System) study is a single-arm, phase-II, multicenter study that enrolled 95 patients with calcified FP lesions less than or equal to 15 cm in length for the evaluation of the Shockwave Lithoplasty treatment. Fig. 3 provides an example of Lithoplasty treatment of a moderately calcified SFA lesion. The Shockwave Lithoplasty treatment is a novel technique that combines interventional delivery of the device and the known lithotripsy applications for disruption of calcium.[97] Pulsatile mechanical energy can disrupt the superficial and deep calcium of the vessel while avoiding tissue injuries. Procedural success (defined by <50% stenosis) was achieved in all the patients, and the average residual stenosis was 23.8%. No

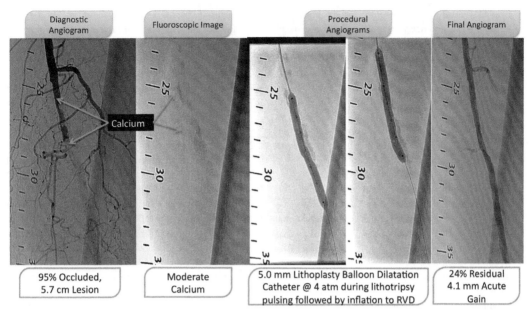

Fig. 3. Peripheral Lithoplasty for treatment of a calcified superficial femoral artery lesion. Baseline angiography shows a moderate to severely calcified distal superficial femoral artery lesion. A 5.0-mm Lithoplasty balloon was inflated during lithotripsy, followed by inflation to the reference vessel diameter (RVD). The final angiogram revealed 24% residual stenosis with a 4.1-mm acute gain. atm, atmospheres. (*Courtesy of* Professor Marianne Brodmann, Graz, Austria.)

amputations, perforations, or distal emboliza-tions were reported at 6-month follow-up, whereas TLR and patency were 3.2% and 76.7% respectively. Shockwave Lithoplasty is FDA cleared and available in Europe since 2015 for patients with PAD calcification. A pro-spective, multicenter, single-blind, randomized (1:1) study that will compare the combination of DCB and the Shockwave Medical Peripheral Lithoplasty System versus DCB alone with con-ventional BA predilation for FP disease with moderate or severe calcification will enroll 300 patients in total (NCT02923193). The safety and effectiveness of Shockwave Lithoplasty will also be assessed for treatment of infrapopliteal disease in 20 patients (NCT02911623).

SUMMARY

Endovascular technologies for PAD have evolved significantly in recent years. However, current treatment options have not eliminated all the disadvantages associated with endovas-cular treatment and newer innovations can generate improved results. Emerging technolo-gies for FP and BTK arteries will provide inter-ventionalists with the ability to intervene on a broader and increasingly complex range of FP and BTK lesions, while maintaining satisfying outcomes and achieving improved rates of acute success and short-term and long-term results for

most of the lesions. Future studies, such as clin-ical trials of advanced-phase and real-world reg-istries, are anticipated to provide continuous surveillance, confirming the effectiveness sug-gested by the initial studies and comparing newer technologies with the established stan-dard of care for endovascular treatment.

REFERENCES

1. Mahoney EM, Wang K, Keo HH, et al. Vascular hospitalization rates and costs in patients with pe-ripheral artery disease in the United States. Circ Cardiovasc Qual Outcomes 2010;3(6):642–51.
2. Fowkes FG, Rudan D, Rudan I, et al. Comparison of global estimates of prevalence and risk factors for peripheral artery disease in 2000 and 2010: a systematic review and analysis. Lancet 2013; 382(9901):1329–40.
3. Singh S, Armstrong EJ, Sherif W, et al. Association of elevated fasting glucose with lower patency and increased major adverse limb events among pa-tients with diabetes undergoing infrapopliteal balloon angioplasty. Vasc Med 2014;19(4):307–14.
4. Westin GG, Armstrong EJ, Bang H, et al. Association between statin medications and mortality, major adverse cardiovascular event, and amputation-free survival in patients with critical limb ischemia. J Am Coll Cardiol 2014;63(7):682–90.
5. Laird JR, Jain A, Zeller T, et al. Nitinol stent implan-tation in the superficial femoral artery and proximal

popliteal artery: twelve-month results from the complete SE multicenter trial. J Endovasc Ther 2014;21(2):202–12.

6. Schillinger M, Sabeti S, Dick P, et al. Sustained benefit at 2 years of primary femoropopliteal stenting compared with balloon angioplasty with optional stenting. Circulation 2007;115(21):2745–9.

7. Axel DI, Kunert W, Goggelmann C, et al. Paclitaxel inhibits arterial smooth muscle cell proliferation and migration in vitro and in vivo using local drug delivery. Circulation 1997;96(2):636–45.

8. Lamichhane S, Anderson J, Remund T, et al. Dextran sulfate as a drug delivery platform for drug-coated balloons: preparation, characterization, in vitro drug elution, and smooth muscle cell response. J Biomed Mater Res B Appl Biomater 2016;104(7):1416–30.

9. Micari A, Cioppa A, Vadala G, et al. Clinical evaluation of a paclitaxel-eluting balloon for treatment of femoropopliteal arterial disease: 12-month results from a multicenter Italian registry. JACC Cardiovasc Interv 2012;5(3):331–8.

10. Tepe G, Laird J, Schneider P, et al. Drug-coated balloon versus standard percutaneous transluminal angioplasty for the treatment of superficial femoral and popliteal peripheral artery disease: 12-month results from the IN.PACT SFA randomized trial. Circulation 2015;131(5):495–502.

11. Rosenfield K, Jaff MR, White CJ, et al. Trial of a paclitaxel-coated balloon for femoropopliteal artery disease. N Engl J Med 2015;373(2):145–53.

12. Micari A, Vadala G, Castriota F, et al. 1-year results of paclitaxel-coated balloons for long femoropopliteal artery disease: evidence from the SFA-long study. JACC Cardiovasc Interv 2016;9(9):950–6.

13. Armstrong EJ, Waldo SW. Drug-coated balloons for long superficial femoral artery disease: leaving nothing behind in the real-world. JACC Cardiovasc Interv 2016;9(9):957–8.

14. Zeller T, Rastan A, Macharzina R, et al. Drug-coated balloons vs. drug-eluting stents for treatment of long femoropopliteal lesions. J Endovasc Ther 2014;21(3):359–68.

15. Bosiers M, Deloose K, Callaert J, et al. Results of the Protege EverFlex 200-mm-long nitinol stent (ev3) in TASC C and D femoropopliteal lesions. J Vasc Surg 2011;54(4):1042–50.

16. Zeller T, Baumgartner I, Scheinert D, et al. Drug-eluting balloon versus standard balloon angioplasty for infrapopliteal arterial revascularization in critical limb ischemia: 12-month results from the IN.PACT DEEP randomized trial. J Am Coll Cardiol 2014;64(15):1568–76.

17. Schmidt A, Piorkowski M, Werner M, et al. First experience with drug-eluting balloons in infrapopliteal arteries: restenosis rate and clinical outcome. J Am Coll Cardiol 2011;58(11):1105–9.

18. Liistro F, Porto I, Angioli P, et al. Drug-eluting Balloon in Peripheral Intervention for Below the Knee Angioplasty Evaluation (DEBATE-BTK): a randomized trial in diabetic patients with critical limb ischemia. Circulation 2013;128(6):615–21.

19. Fanelli F, Cannavale A, Boatta E, et al. Lower limb multilevel treatment with drug-eluting balloons: 6-month results from the DEBELLUM randomized trial. J Endovasc Ther 2012;19(5):571–80.

20. Zeller T, Beschorner U, Pilger E, et al. Paclitaxel-coated balloon in infrapopliteal arteries: 12-month results from the BIOLUX P-II randomized trial (BIOTRONIK'S-First in Man study of the Passeo-18 LUX drug releasing PTA balloon catheter vs. the uncoated Passeo-18 PTA balloon catheter in subjects requiring revascularization of infrapopliteal arteries). JACC Cardiovasc Interv 2015;8(12):1614–22.

21. Steiner S, Schmidt A, Bausback Y, et al. Single-center experience with Lutonix drug-coated balloons in infrapopliteal arteries. J Endovasc Ther 2016;23(3):417–23.

22. Schroeder H, Meyer DR, Lux B, et al. Two-year results of a low-dose drug-coated balloon for revascularization of the femoropopliteal artery: outcomes from the ILLUMENATE first-in-human study. Catheter Cardiovasc Interv 2015;86(2):278–86.

23. Perez de Prado A, Perez-Martinez C, Cuellas Ramon C, et al. Safety and efficacy of different paclitaxel-eluting balloons in a porcine model. Rev Esp Cardiol (Engl Ed) 2014;67(6):456–62.

24. Schillinger M, Sabeti S, Loewe C, et al. Balloon angioplasty versus implantation of nitinol stents in the superficial femoral artery. N Engl J Med 2006;354(18):1879–88.

25. Scheinert D, Scheinert S, Sax J, et al. Prevalence and clinical impact of stent fractures after femoropopliteal stenting. J Am Coll Cardiol 2005;45(2):312–5.

26. Schlager O, Dick P, Sabeti S, et al. Long-segment SFA stenting–the dark sides: in-stent restenosis, clinical deterioration, and stent fractures. J Endovasc Ther 2005;12(6):676–84.

27. Klein AJ, Chen SJ, Messenger JC, et al. Quantitative assessment of the conformational change in the femoropopliteal artery with leg movement. Catheter Cardiovasc Interv 2009;74(5):787–98.

28. Laird JR. Limitations of percutaneous transluminal angioplasty and stenting for the treatment of disease of the superficial femoral and popliteal arteries. J Endovasc Ther 2006;13(Suppl 2):Ii30–40.

29. Dake MD, Ansel GM, Jaff MR, et al. Sustained safety and effectiveness of paclitaxel-eluting stents for femoropopliteal lesions: 2-year follow-up from the Zilver PTX randomized and single-arm clinical studies. J Am Coll Cardiol 2013;61(24):2417–27.

30. Dake MD, Ansel GM, Jaff MR, et al. Durable clinical effectiveness with paclitaxel-eluting stents in the femoropopliteal artery: 5-year results of the Zilver

PTX randomized trial. Circulation 2016;133(15): 1472–83 [discussion: 1483].

31. Yokoi H, Ohki T, Kichikawa K, et al. Zilver PTX post-market surveillance study of paclitaxel-eluting stents for treating femoropopliteal artery disease in Japan: 12-month results. JACC Cardiovasc Interv 2016;9(3):271–7.

32. Conrad MF, Crawford RS, Hackney LA, et al. Endo-vascular management of patients with critical limb ischemia. J Vasc Surg 2011;53(4):1020–5.

33. Gandini R, Volpi T, Pampana E, et al. Applicability and clinical results of percutaneous transluminal angioplasty with a novel, long, conically shaped balloon dedicated for below-the knee interventions. J Cardiovasc Surg 2009;50(3):365–71.

34. Spiliopoulos S, Theodosiadou V, Katsanos K, et al. Long-term clinical outcomes of infrapopliteal drug-eluting stent placement for critical limb ischemia in diabetic patients. J Vasc Interv Radiol 2015;26(10): 1423–30.

35. Fusaro M, Cassese S, Ndrepepa G, et al. Drug-eluting stents for revascularization of infrapopliteal arteries: updated meta-analysis of randomized trials. JACC Cardiovasc Interv 2013;6(12):1284–93.

36. Spreen MI, Martens JM, Hansen BE, et al. Percuta-neous transluminal angioplasty and drug-eluting stents for infrapopliteal lesions in critical limb ischemia (PADI) trial. Circ Cardiovasc Interv 2016;9(2):e002376.

37. Scheinert D, Katsanos K, Zeller T, et al. A prospective randomized multicenter comparison of balloon an-gioplasty and infrapopliteal stenting with the sirolimus-eluting stent in patients with ischemic pe-ripheral arterial disease: 1-year results from the ACHILLES trial. J Am Coll Cardiol 2012;60(22):2290–5.

38. Bosiers M, Scheinert D, Peeters P, et al. Random-ized comparison of everolimus-eluting versus bare-metal stents in patients with critical limb ischemia and infrapopliteal arterial occlusive dis-ease. J Vasc Surg 2012;55(2):390–8.

39. Rastan A, Brechtel K, Krankenberg H, et al. Siroli-mus-eluting stents for treatment of infrapopliteal arteries reduce clinical event rate compared to bare-metal stents: long-term results from a ran-domized trial. J Am Coll Cardiol 2012;60(7):587–91.

40. Siablis D, Kitrou PM, Spiliopoulos S, et al. Pacli-taxel-coated balloon angioplasty versus drug-eluting stenting for the treatment of infrapopliteal long-segment arterial occlusive disease: the IDEAS randomized controlled trial. JACC Cardiovasc Interv 2014;7(9):1048–56.

41. Hou D, Huibregtse BA, Eppihimer M, et al. Fluoro-copolymer-coated nitinol self-expanding pacli-taxel-eluting stent: pharmacokinetics and vascular biology responses in a porcine iliofemoral model. EuroIntervention 2016;12(6):790–7.

42. Muller-Hulsbeck S, Keirse K, Zeller T, et al. Twelve-month results from the MAJESTIC trial of the Eluvia

paclitaxel-eluting stent for treatment of obstructive femoropopliteal disease. J Endovasc Ther 2016; 23(5):701–7.

43. Patel N, Banning AP. Bioabsorbable scaffolds for the treatment of obstructive coronary artery dis-ease: the next revolution in coronary intervention? Heart 2013;99(17):1236–43.

44. Karnabatidis D, Katsanos K, Spiliopoulos S, et al. Incidence, anatomical location, and clinical signifi-cance of compressions and fractures in infrapopli-teal balloon-expandable metal stents. J Endovasc Ther 2009;16(1):15–22.

45. Neil N. Stent fracture in the superficial femoral and proximal popliteal arteries: literature summary and economic impacts. Perspect Vasc Surg Endovasc Ther 2013;25(1–2):20–7.

46. Bosiers M, Peeters P, D'Archambeau O, et al. AMS INSIGHT–absorbable metal stent implantation for treatment of below-the-knee critical limb ischemia: 6-month analysis. Cardiovasc Intervent Radiol 2009; 32(3):424–35.

47. Bosiers M, Deloose K, Verbist J, et al. First clinical application of absorbable metal stents in the treat-ment of critical limb ischemia: 12-month results VASCULAR DISEASE MANAGEMENT2008. 2016. Available at: http://www.vasculardiseasemanage-ment.com/article/4362. Accessed February 11, 2016.

48. Bontinck J, Goverde P, Schroe H, et al. Treatment of the femoropopliteal artery with the bioresorbable REMEDY stent. J Vasc Surg 2016;64(5):1311–9.

49. Werner M, Schmidt A, Scheinert S, et al. Evaluation of the biodegradable Igaki-Tamai scaffold after drug-eluting balloon treatment of de novo superfi-cial femoral artery lesions: the GAIA-DEB study. J Endovasc Ther 2016;23(1):92–7.

50. Peeters P, Bosiers M, Verbist J, et al. Preliminary re-sults after application of absorbable metal stents in patients with critical limb ischemia. J Endovasc Ther 2005;12(1):1–5.

51. Di Mario C, Griffiths H, Goktekin O, et al. Drug-eluting bioabsorbable magnesium stent. J Interv Cardiol 2004;17(6):391–5.

52. Varcoe RL, Schouten O, Thomas SD, et al. Initial experience with the Absorb bioresorbable vascular scaffold below the knee: six-month clinical and imag-ing outcomes. J Endovasc Ther 2015;22(2):226–32.

53. Karanian JW, Peregoy JA, Chiesa OA, et al. Effi-ciency of drug delivery to the coronary arteries in swine is dependent on the route of administration: assessment of luminal, intimal, and adventitial cor-onary artery and venous delivery methods. J Vasc Interv Radiol 2010;21(10):1555–64.

54. Wilcox JN, Waksman R, King SB, et al. The role of the adventitia in the arterial response to angio-plasty: the effect of intravascular radiation. Int J Radiat Oncol Biol Phys 1996;36(4):789–96.

55. Scott NA, Cipolla GD, Ross CE, et al. Identification of a potential role for the adventitia in vascular lesion formation after balloon overstretch injury of porcine coronary arteries. Circulation 1996;93(12):2178–87.

56. Siow RC, Mallawaarachchi CM, Weissberg PL. Migration of adventitial myofibroblasts following vascular balloon injury: insights from in vivo gene transfer to rat carotid arteries. Cardiovasc Res 2003;59(1):212–21.

57. Okamoto E, Couse T, De Leon H, et al. Perivascular inflammation after balloon angioplasty of porcine coronary arteries. Circulation 2001;104(18):2228–35.

58. Maiellaro K, Taylor WR. The role of the adventitia in vascular inflammation. Cardiovasc Res 2007;75(4):640–8.

59. Hu Y, Xu Q. Adventitial biology: differentiation and function. Arterioscler Thromb Vasc Biol 2011;31(7):1523–9.

60. Owens CD, Gasper WJ, Walker JP, et al. Safety and feasibility of adjunctive dexamethasone infusion into the adventitia of the femoropopliteal artery following endovascular revascularization. J Vasc Surg 2014;59(4):1016–24.

61. Gasper WJ, Jimenez CA, Walker J, et al. Adventitial nab-rapamycin injection reduces porcine femoral artery luminal stenosis induced by balloon angioplasty via inhibition of medial proliferation and adventitial inflammation. Circ Cardiovasc Interv 2013;6(6):701–9.

62. Burke SK, Macdonald K, Moss E, et al. Effects of recombinant human type I pancreatic elastase on human atherosclerotic arteries. J Cardiovasc Pharmacol 2014;64(6):530–5.

63. Coen M, Gabbiani G, Bochaton-Piallat ML. Myofibroblast-mediated adventitial remodeling: an underestimated player in arterial pathology. Arterioscler Thromb Vasc Biol 2011;31(11):2391–6.

64. Mecham RP, Broekelmann TJ, Fliszar CJ, et al. Elastin degradation by matrix metalloproteinases. Cleavage site specificity and mechanisms of elastolysis. J Biol Chem 1997;272(29):18071–6.

65. Qamar AA, Burke SK, Lafleur JD, et al. The ability of serum from alpha 1-antitrypsin-deficient patients to inhibit PRT-201, a recombinant human type I pancreatic elastase. Biotechnol Appl Biochem 2012;59(1):22–8.

66. Dwivedi AJ, Roy-Chaudhury P, Peden EK, et al. Application of human type I pancreatic elastase (PRT-201) to the venous anastomosis of arteriovenous grafts in patients with chronic kidney disease. J Vasc Access 2014;15(5):376–84.

67. Hye RJ, Peden EK, O'Connor TP, et al. Human type I pancreatic elastase treatment of arteriovenous fistulas in patients with chronic kidney disease. J Vasc Surg 2014;60(2):454–61.e1.

68. Peden EK, Leeser DB, Dixon BS, et al. A multi-center, dose-escalation study of human type I pancreatic elastase (PRT-201) administered after arteriovenous fistula creation. J Vasc Access 2013;14(2):143–51.

69. Tepe G, Zeller T, Schnorr B, et al. High-grade, non-flow-limiting dissections do not negatively impact long-term outcome after paclitaxel-coated balloon angioplasty: an additional analysis from the THUNDER study. J Endovasc Ther 2013;20(6):792–800.

70. Werk M, Albrecht T, Meyer DR, et al. Paclitaxel-coated balloons reduce restenosis after femoropopliteal angioplasty: evidence from the randomized PACIFIER trial. Circ Cardiovasc Interv 2012;5(6):831–40.

71. Tepe G, Zeller T, Albrecht T, et al. Local delivery of paclitaxel to inhibit restenosis during angioplasty of the leg. N Engl J Med 2008;358(7):689–99.

72. Tosaka A, Soga Y, Iida O, et al. Classification and clinical impact of restenosis after femoropopliteal stenting. J Am Coll Cardiol 2012;59(1):16–23.

73. Kiguchi MM, Marone LK, Chaer RA, et al. Patterns of femoropopliteal recurrence after routine and selective stenting endoluminal therapy. J Vasc Surg 2013;57(1):37–43.

74. Schneider PA, Giasolli R, Ebner A, et al. Early experimental and clinical experience with a focal implant for lower extremity post-angioplasty dissection. JACC Cardiovasc Interv 2015;8(2):347–54.

75. Bosiers M, Scheinert D, Hendriks JM, et al. Results from the Tack Optimized Balloon Angioplasty (TOBA) study demonstrate the benefits of minimal metal implants for dissection repair after angioplasty. J Vasc Surg 2016;64(1):109–16.

76. David Smith C, Gavin Bilmen J, Iqbal S, et al. Medial artery calcification as an indicator of diabetic peripheral vascular disease. Foot Ankle Int 2008;29(2):185–90.

77. Bishop PD, Feiten LE, Ouriel K, et al. Arterial calcification increases in distal arteries in patients with peripheral arterial disease. Ann Vasc Surg 2008;22(6):799–805.

78. Pohle K, Maffert R, Ropers D, et al. Progression of aortic valve calcification: association with coronary atherosclerosis and cardiovascular risk factors. Circulation 2001;104(16):1927–32.

79. Rennenberg RJ, Kessels AG, Schurgers LJ, et al. Vascular calcifications as a marker of increased cardiovascular risk: a meta-analysis. Vasc Health Risk Manag 2009;5(1):185–97.

80. Huang CL, Wu IH, Wu YW, et al. Association of lower extremity arterial calcification with amputation and mortality in patients with symptomatic peripheral artery disease. PLoS One 2014;9(2):e90201.

81. Spaargaren GJ, Lee MJ, Reekers JA, et al. Evaluation of a new balloon catheter for difficult calcified lesions in infrainguinal arterial disease: outcome of a multicenter registry. Cardiovasc Intervent Radiol 2009;32(1):132–5.

82. Shammas NW, Coiner D, Shammas G, et al. Predictors of provisional stenting in patients undergoing lower extremity arterial interventions. Int J Angiol 2011;20(2):95–100.

83. Cheng CP, Choi G, Herfkens RJ, et al. The effect of aging on deformations of the superficial femoral artery resulting from hip and knee flexion: potential clinical implications. J Vasc Interv Radiol 2010; 21(2):195–202.

84. Otsuka Y, Kasahara Y, Kawamura A. Use of SafeCut Balloon for treatment of in-stent restenosis of a previously underexpanded sirolimus-eluting stent with a heavily calcified plaque. J Invasive Cardiol 2007;19(12):E359–62.

85. Feldman DN. Atherectomy for calcified femoropopliteal disease: are we making progress? J Invasive Cardiol 2014;26(8):304–6.

86. Lee MS, Canan T, Rha SW, et al. Pooled analysis of the CONFIRM registries: impact of gender on procedure and angiographic outcomes in patients undergoing orbital atherectomy for peripheral artery disease. J Endovasc Ther 2015;22(1):57–62.

87. Shammas NW, Lam R, Mustapha J, et al. Comparison of orbital atherectomy plus balloon angioplasty vs. balloon angioplasty alone in patients with critical limb ischemia: results of the CALCIUM 360 randomized pilot trial. J Endovasc Ther 2012;19(4):480–8.

88. Korabathina R, Mody KP, Yu J, et al. Orbital atherectomy for symptomatic lower extremity disease. Catheter Cardiovasc Interv 2010;76(3):326–32.

89. Minko P, Katoh M, Jaeger S, et al. Atherectomy of heavily calcified femoropopliteal stenotic lesions. J Vasc Interv Radiol 2011;22(7):995–1000.

90. Sixt S, Rastan A, Scheinert D, et al. The 1-year clinical impact of rotational aspiration atherectomy of infrainguinal lesions. Angiology 2011;62(8):645–56.

91. Banerjee A, Sarode K, Mohammad A, et al. Safety and effectiveness of the Nav-6 filter in preventing distal embolization during Jetstream atherectomy of infrainguinal peripheral artery lesions. J Invasive Cardiol 2016;28(8):330–3.

92. Shammas NW, Shammas GA, Banerjee S, et al. JetStream rotational and aspiration atherectomy in treating in-stent restenosis of the femoropopliteal arteries: results of the JETSTREAM-ISR feasibility study. J Endovasc Ther 2016;23(2): 339–46.

93. Dave RM, Patlola R, Kollmeyer K, et al. Excimer laser recanalization of femoropopliteal lesions and 1-year patency: results of the CELLO registry. J Endovasc Ther 2009;16(6):665–75.

94. Cioppa A, Stabile E, Popusoi G, et al. Combined treatment of heavy calcified femoro-popliteal lesions using directional atherectomy and a paclitaxel coated balloon: one-year single centre clinical results. Cardiovasc Revasc Med 2012;13(4): 219–23.

95. Khalid MR, Khalid FR, Farooqui FA, et al. A novel catheter in patients with peripheral chronic total occlusions: a single center experience. Catheter Cardiovasc Interv 2010;76(5):735–9.

96. Ichihashi S, Sato T, Iwakoshi S, et al. Technique of percutaneous direct needle puncture of calcified plaque in the superficial femoral artery or tibial artery to facilitate balloon catheter passage and balloon dilation of calcified lesions. J Vasc Interv Radiol 2014;25(5):784–8.

97. Damianou C, Couppis A. Feasibility study for removing calcified material using a planar rectangular ultrasound transducer. J Ultrasound 2016; 19(2):115–23.

98. Varcoe RL, Schouten O, Thomas SD, et al. Experience with the absorb everolimus-eluting bioresorbable vascular scaffold in arteries below the knee: 12-month clinical and imaging outcomes. JACC Cardiovasc Interv 2016;9(16):1721–8.

Moving?

Make sure your subscription moves with you!

To notify us of your new address, find your **Clinics Account Number** (located on your mailing label above your name), and contact customer service at:

Email: journalscustomerservice-usa@elsevier.com

800-654-2452 (subscribers in the U.S. & Canada)
314-447-8871 (subscribers outside of the U.S. & Canada)

Fax number: 314-447-8029

Elsevier Health Sciences Division
Subscription Customer Service
3251 Riverport Lane
Maryland Heights, MO 63043

Printed and bound by CPI Group (UK) Ltd, Croydon, CR0 4YY

03/10/2024

01040385-0003